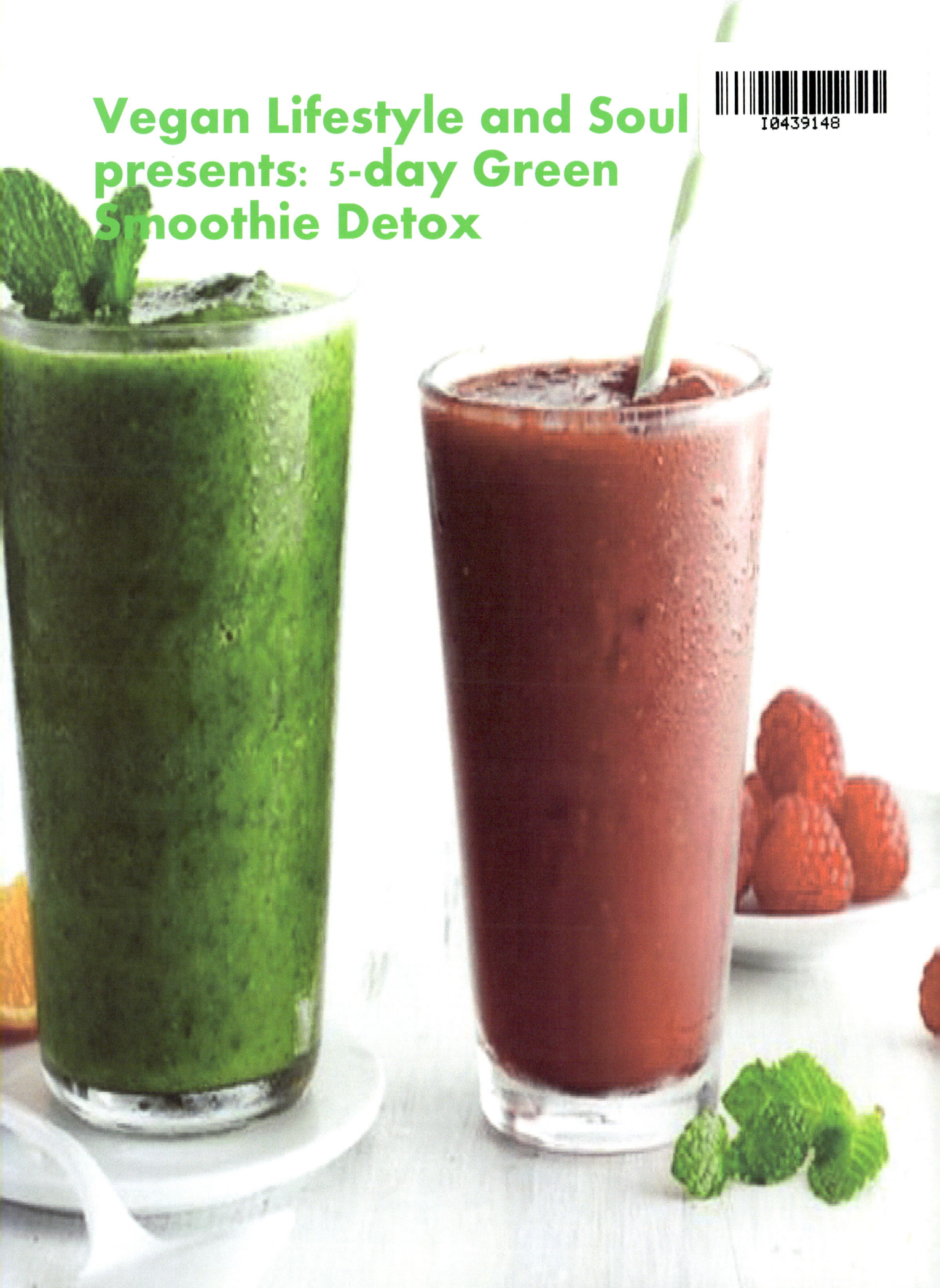

Vegan Lifestyle and Soul presents: 5-day Green Smoothie Detox

Table of Contents

INTRODUCTION

There are many symptoms which should ring alarms for you to take the detoxification programs. A change in routine and diet can bring along multiple long-lasting benefits for your body which has been badly affected by toxins. Proteins, minerals and vitamins found in different fruits, vegetables and other foods are essential for your body and the detox programs help you in taking sufficient amounts of these along with enough physical exercise. In many cases, this might be the only solution to headaches, irritation, extreme food cravings and unwanted pounds. To your surprise, controlling your habits can actually make you fit into your jeans in only a few days!

WHAT IS DETOXIFICATION

Before we move on to anything, we need to know what detoxification really is. Detoxification is one of the processes carried out in your body naturally in order to neutralize or get rid of unnecessary or harmful toxins. This is one of the fundamental processes that are continuously going on in your body to keep you healthy. The function also interacts with other parts of your body. So this means that detoxification is all about improving a particular function of your body. Detoxification has two sections. One, reducing the amount of toxins we take in; and second, boosting the processes by intake of important nutrients.

Important Notice - Consult your physician before starting any diet, exercise, or nutritional supplement program.

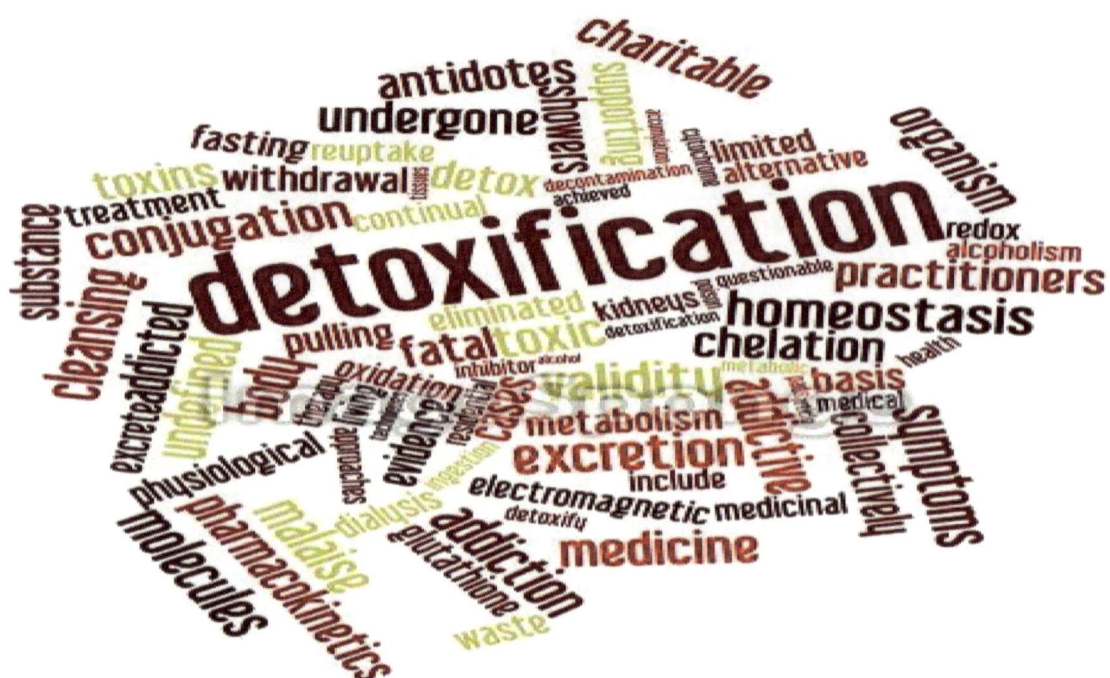

TYPES OF DETOXIFICATION

Alcohol Detoxification

Extreme alcohol addiction may result in down-regulation of GABA neurotransmitter receptors in our body. Through the process of alcohol detoxification, the internal systems of such addicts are brought back to normal.

However, alcohol detoxification is not the only solution for withdrawal of alcohol. The addict might face extreme, lethal effects if proper medical treatment is not given after detoxification. Even though detoxification is essential, alcoholism requires medical management and other treatments to be treated.

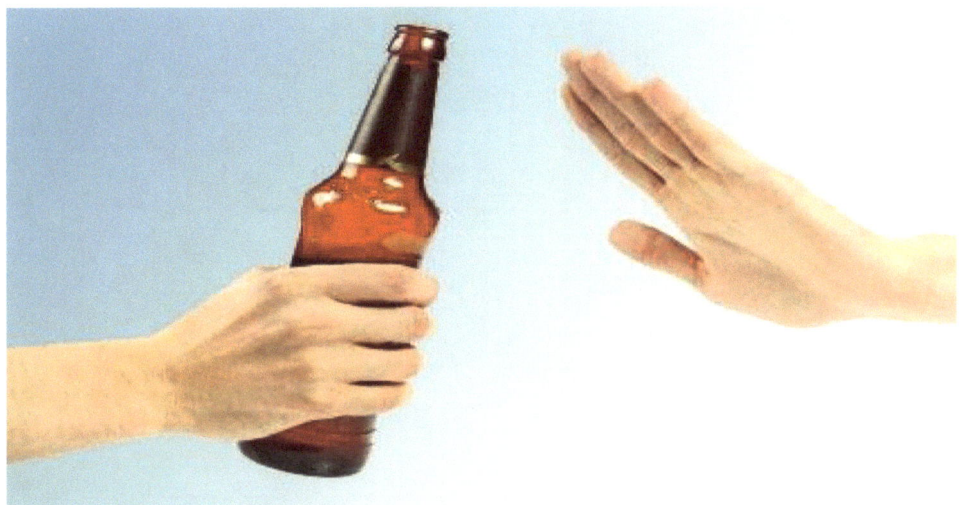

Drug Detoxification

Just like alcohol detoxification, drug detoxification has been chosen by doctors to minimize the withdrawal systems on a drug addict in order to make the process easier. Drug detoxification is not a solution for drug addiction; it rather makes the medical treatment of drug addicts less challenging. Drug detoxification is an early step to a following long term medical treatment. Drug detoxification can be done with medications and can last for few months; however, the process mainly takes place in your house rather than a medical clinic.

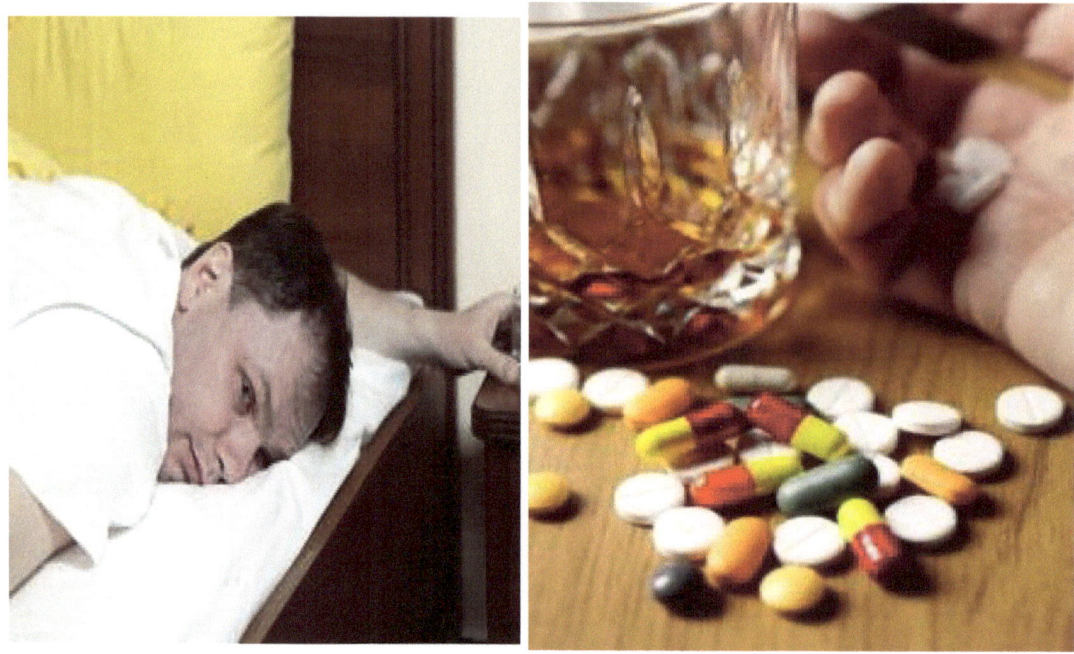

The process of drug detoxification can vary according to the treatment location, however the main purpose remains the same; providing treatment in order to avoid mental and physical symptoms following the withdrawal of alcohol and other drugs.

Metabolic Detoxification

The metabolism in animals produces harmful and toxic substances. They need to be made less harmful through the redox reactions (oxidation and reduction), and combination or excretion of these toxins from tissues or cells. This is known as xenobiotic metabolism. Certain enzymes in the body are essential in the process of detoxification metabolism. These include glutathione S-transferases, cytochrome P450 oxidases, and UDP-glucuronosyltransferases.

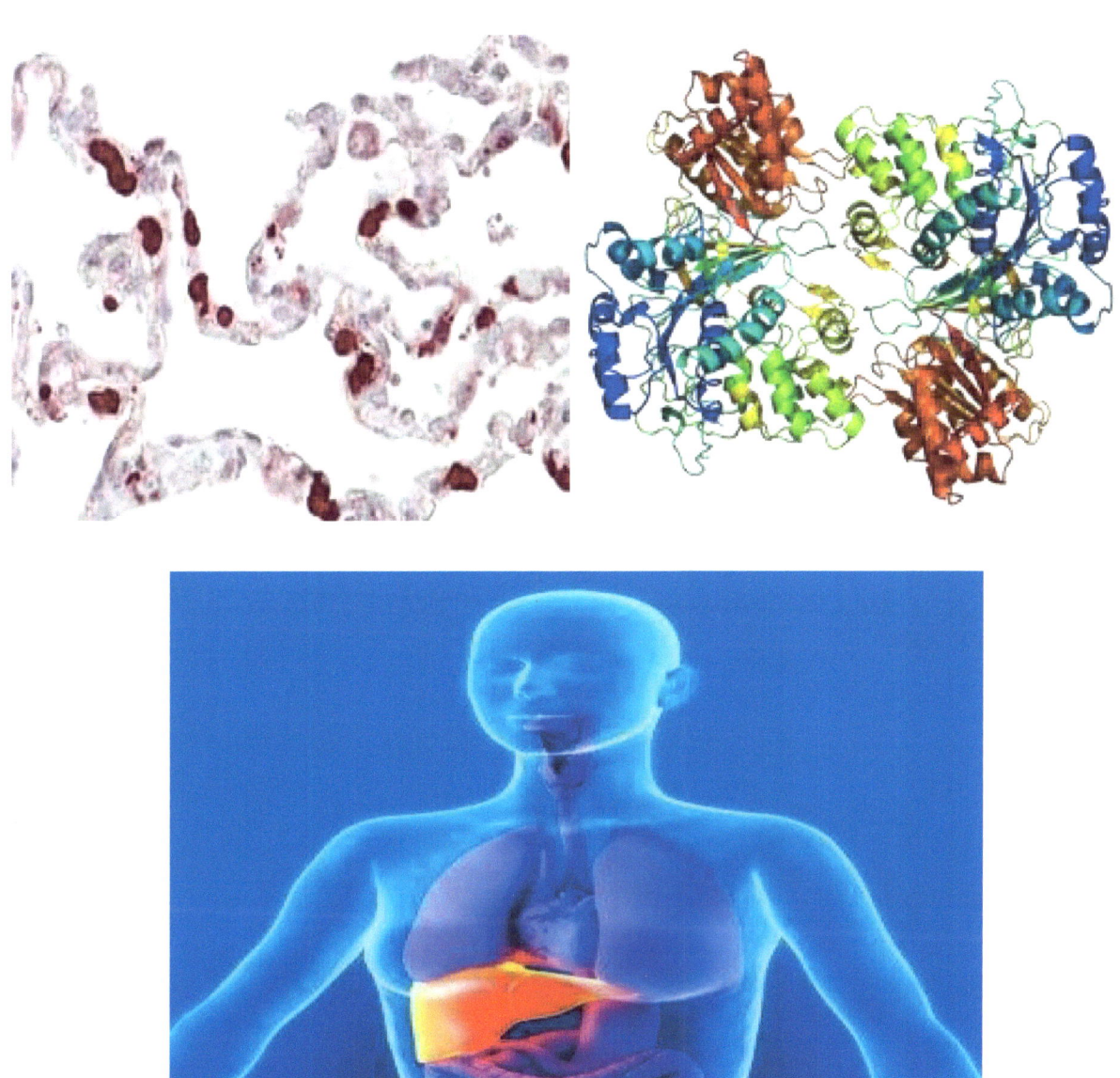

Liver and Internal Cleaning:

Almost all of us understand what cleanliness of the body means. Cleaning your teeth twice a day, taking showers and washing your hair are a few examples of our everyday chores in order to keep ourselves clean. However, what we don't really know is that there is more that our body needs than just washing or cleaning our outer selves. The body needs some cleaning internally too, and this is why it carries out the process of detoxification. The problem, however, is that we never know when our body needs this cleaning more than it normally would. When you're sweating, you know that your body needs a shower. But it's very difficult to find out that your body needs some filtration inside.

The liver is the main organ that carries out this process. It filters the toxins and bacteria in our blood and converts them into elements or substances which can be eliminated by kidneys. So, it's hard to find out when this mechanism isn't working well and our liver needs some boost. Detoxification is a key mechanism of body that needs help from hundreds of molecules in our bodies that are manufactured every day. Our bodies need a very large number of enzymes, minerals, vitamins, and other substances to clean our bodies by getting free of, or transforming the toxins and waste products in our bodies.. However, the process of detoxification is not as simple as it seems. Even though the liver is the main organ responsible for this function, the kidneys, skin, lymphatic system and lungs, all play their roles in cleansing of your body. Hence, the enzymes and molecules which basically carry out the process need to be manufactured first so that the overall process is improved.

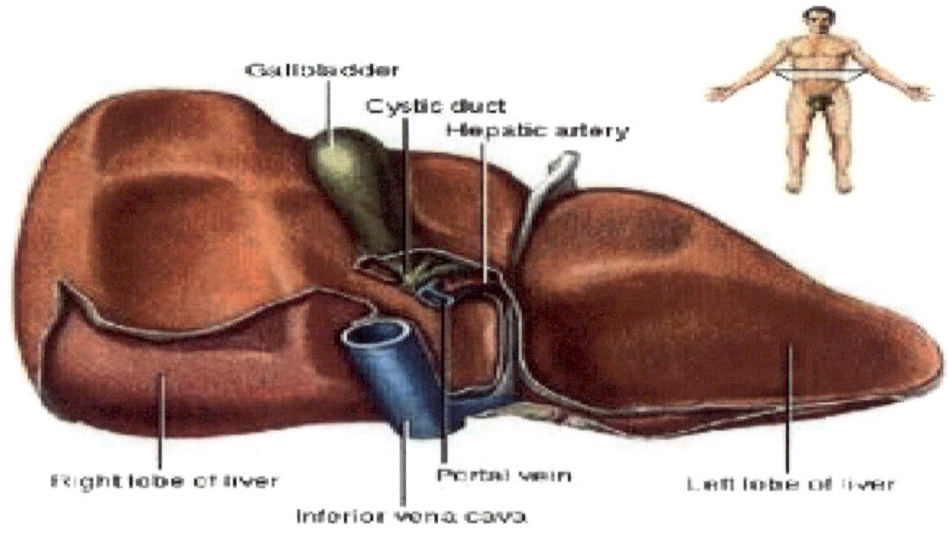

THE DETOXIFICATION PROGRAM

The purpose of the detoxification process would now be clear to you; it is to trigger the main organs so that your body metabolizes and excretes the unwanted toxins in the body. Linda Page, ND, PhD, a lecturer, naturopathic doctor, author of the book *Detoxification* has said, "It's a way to recharge, rejuvenate, and renew. Anybody can benefit from a cleansing. It's a way you can jump-start your body for a more active life, a healthier life."

No matter how complex the process is in your bodies, it can be very simple for you; just follow a routine intake of some particular vegetables, fruits and other minerals. With a little determination and persistence, you can help yourself rehabilitate and get rid of the harmful toxins inside your body through simple steps towards detoxification. This enables you to stay healthier, happier and more energetic.

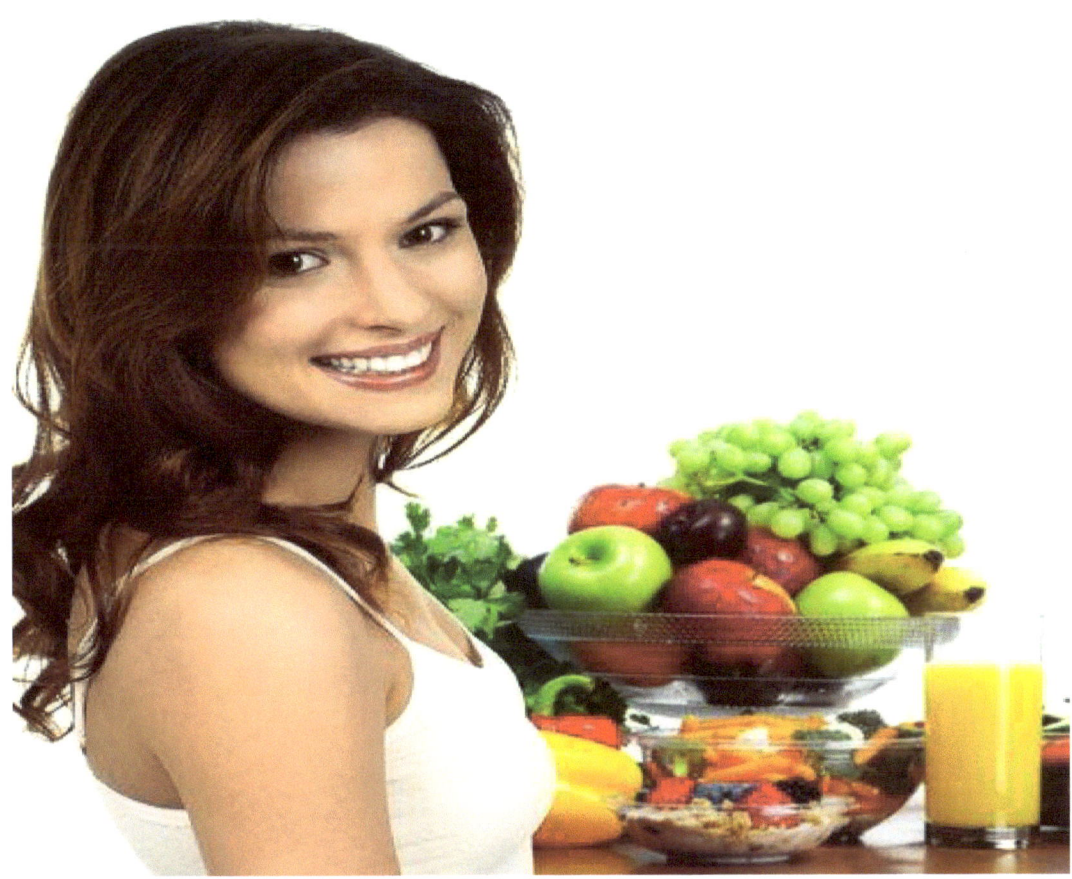

LONG-TERM AND SHORT-TERM DETOX

Detoxification programs can be long-term or short-term depending upon the requirement of your body but they both have the same purpose of removing unwanted substances from the body.

<u>Short-term detoxification</u> includes:

- Chelation Therapy

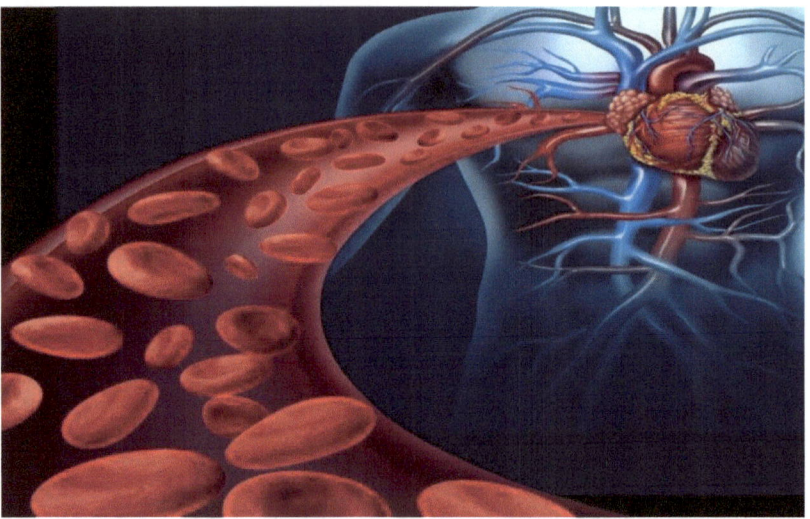

- colon cleansing

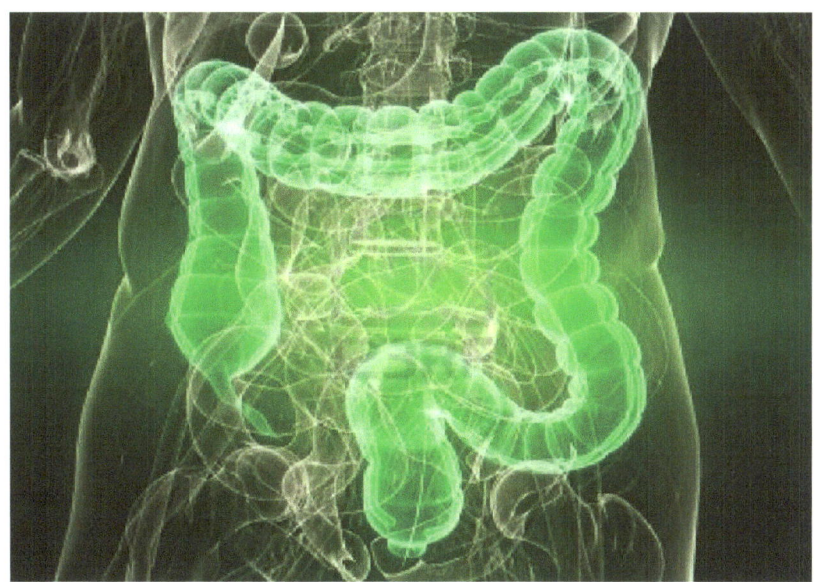

- safe mercury removal

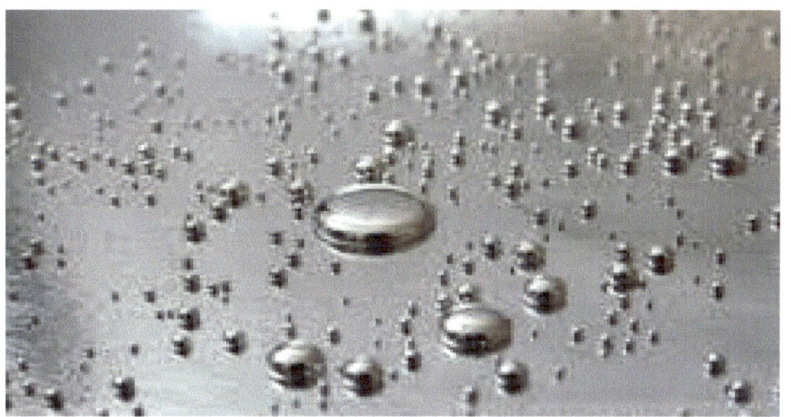

- heavy metal removal

- skin cleansing

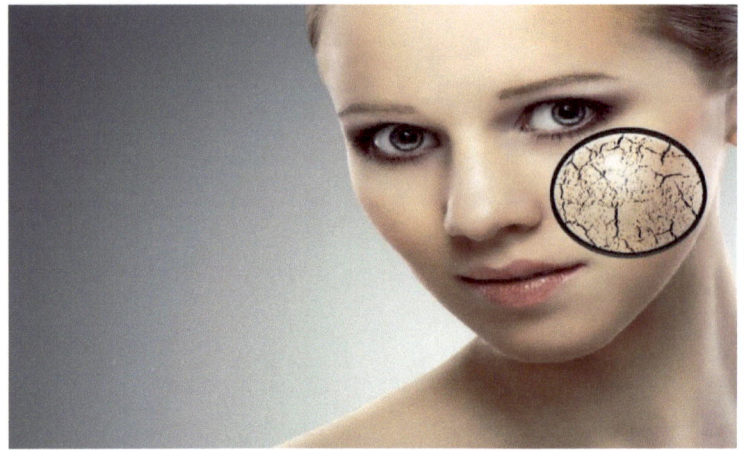

- 24-hour juice fasting

- intravenous injections

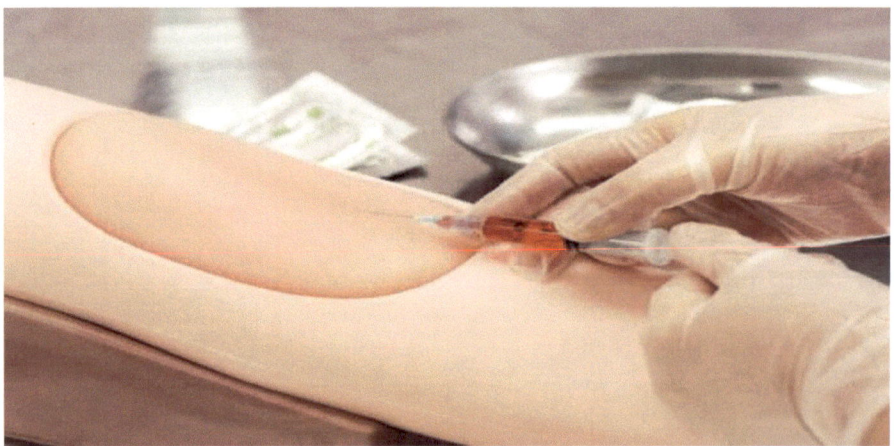

Long-term detoxification is different and the results are obviously not very obvious. It requires many dietary changes. You have to change your eating habits so that a good result can be seen in the long run. Long term detoxification may also require you to do certain exercises regularly. Long-term detox programs may require you to:

- Avoid high carbs and sweeteners

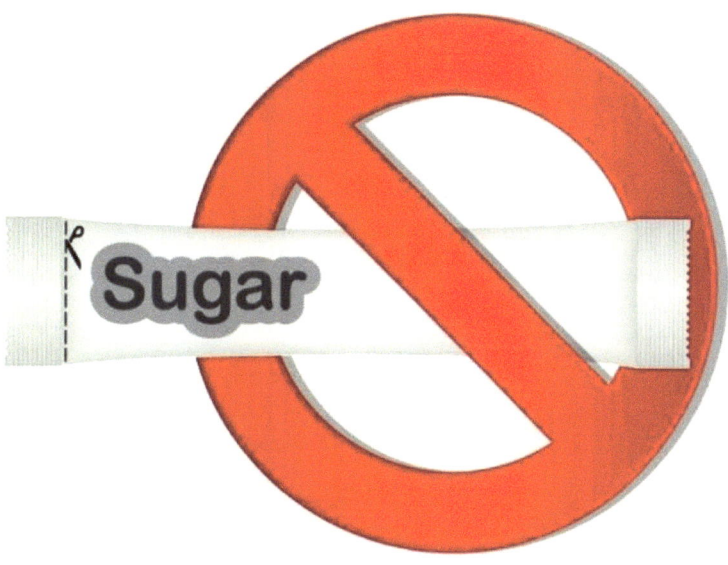

- Add sufficient quantities of fruits and vegetables to your diet

- Avoid meats

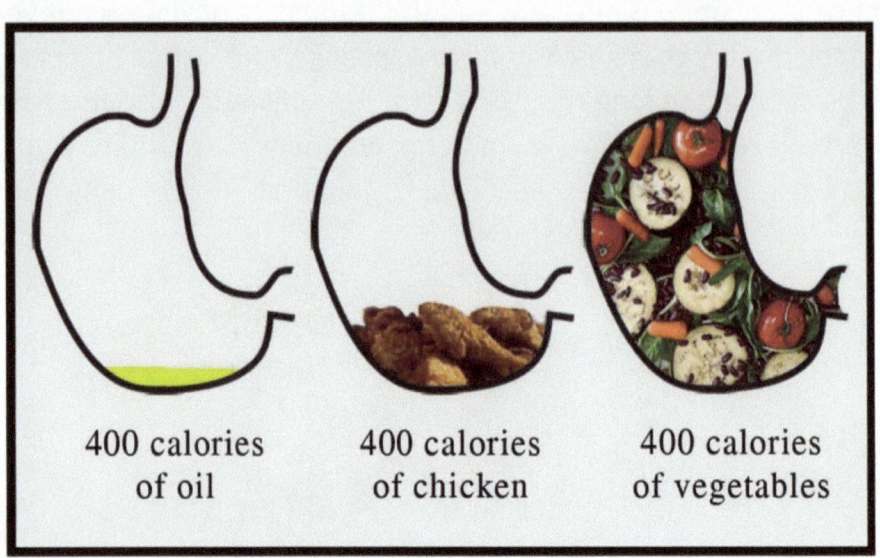

400 calories of oil   400 calories of chicken   400 calories of vegetables

- Drink more juices or fluids, such as herbal tea, water, or vegetable and fruit juice

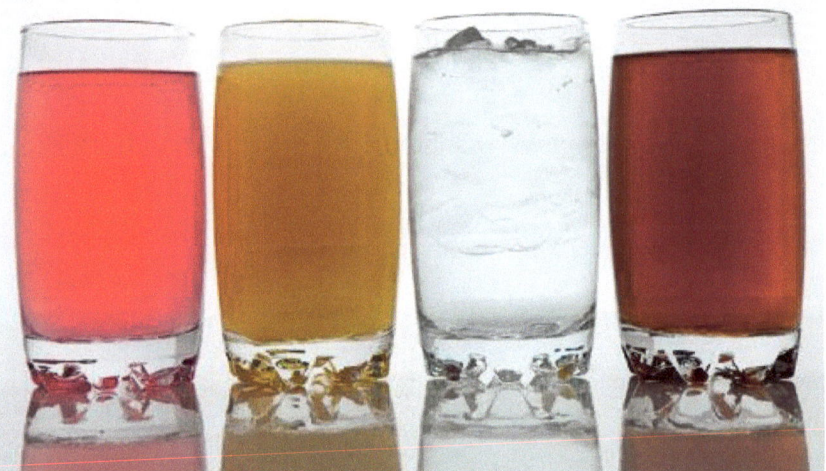

- Eat foods with more vitamins and proteins

- Do exercises like yoga regularly

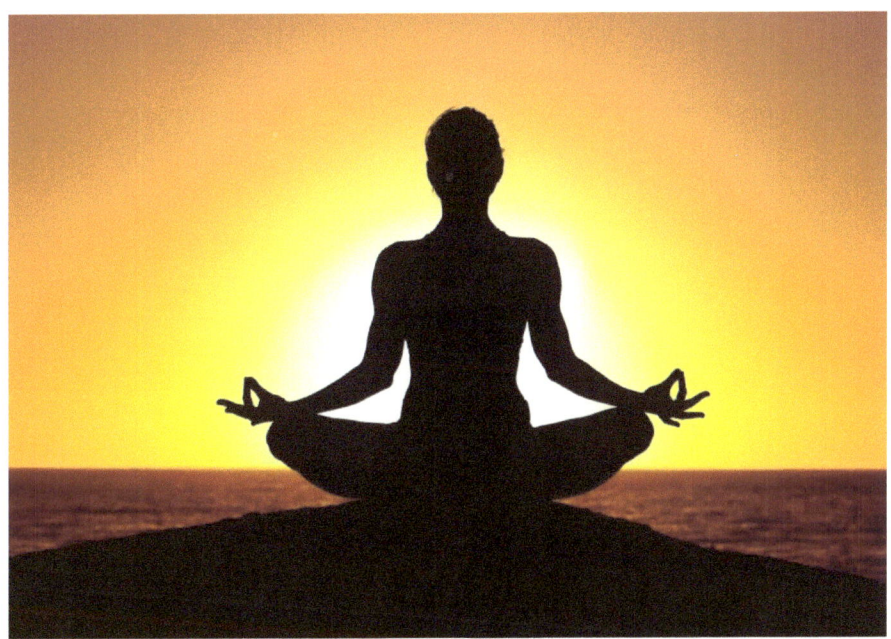

- Try stress-releasing methods like meditation, herbal soaks and massage

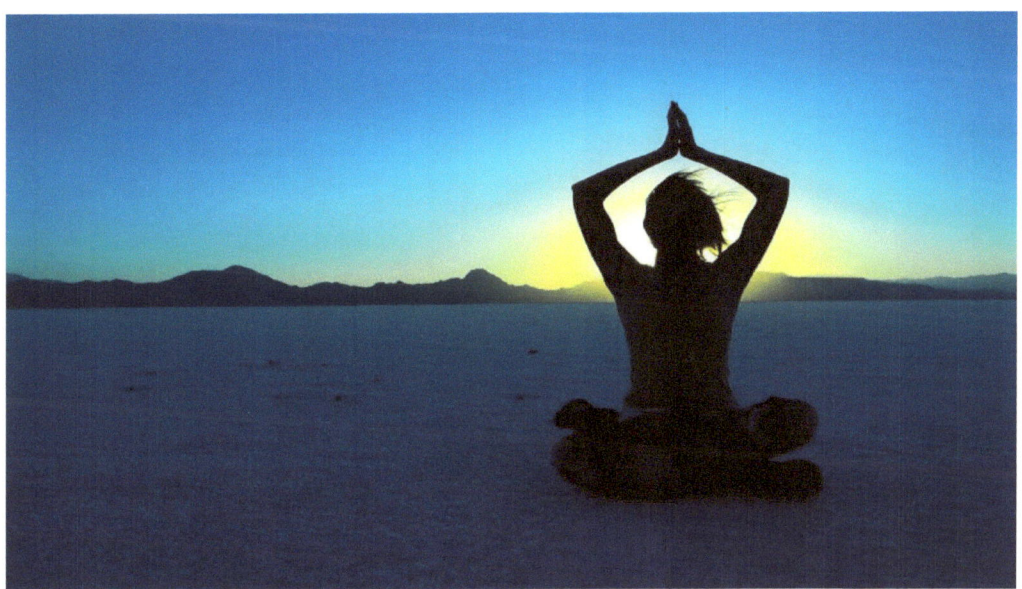

- Try other therapies like acupuncture, homeopathy and hydrotherapy.

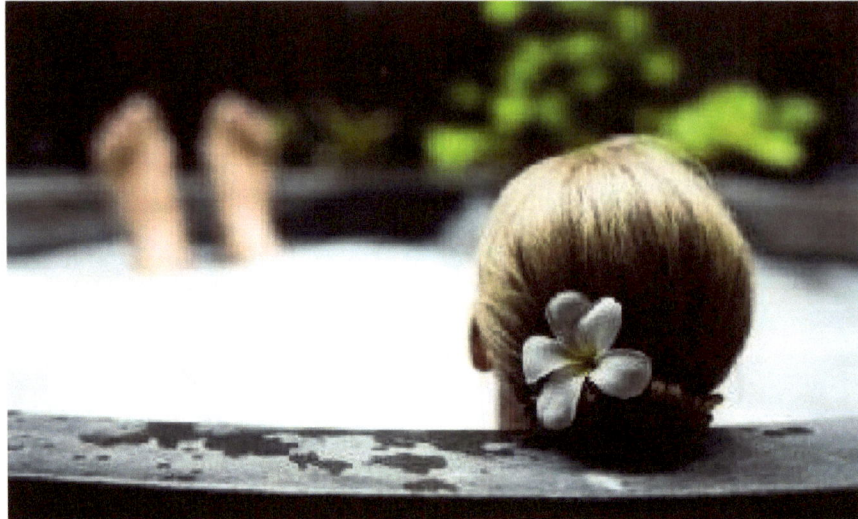

WHY DETOXIFICATION?

FLC (Feel Like Crap) Syndrome

Toxic substances in the body make you feel like vibrant and active. No matter how many hours of sleep you get, when you wake up you do not appear energetic, joyful or vital. The toxics in your body can actually take away all the joy and happiness of your life. It can even make thin people sense symptoms of being toxic like achiness, allergies, brain fog, fatigue, headaches, migraines, and digestion problems. This is when detoxification can come to your rescue. You might have to keep a control on your diet, but it's just a matter of few days until you start feeling all good again.

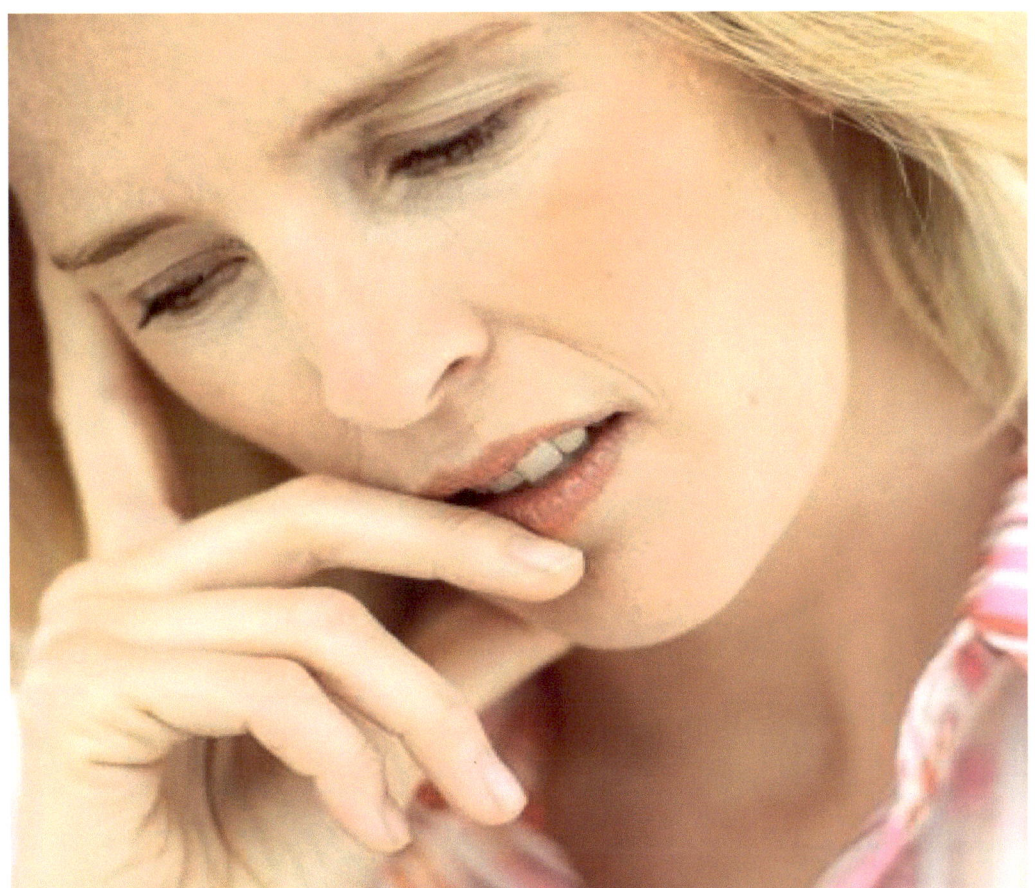

Diet and exercise are not the everything for weight loss

We have been convinced through science that our weight is the exchange of calories in and out of our system. This leads us to the conclusion less eating and more exercise is the way to reduce our weight. However, this is not quite true and not as effective as one might think. The key behind understanding our system of weights is elimination and identification. Through established science for diet, we know that sugar calories are actually quite different from other calories. They aren't the same as other calories because they are the root cause of the trigger for overeating and addiction. They cause inflammation and this gives us the feeling of being hungry. Conclusively, the first and foremost aspect of your weight loss is that sugar calories need to be eliminated from our diet.

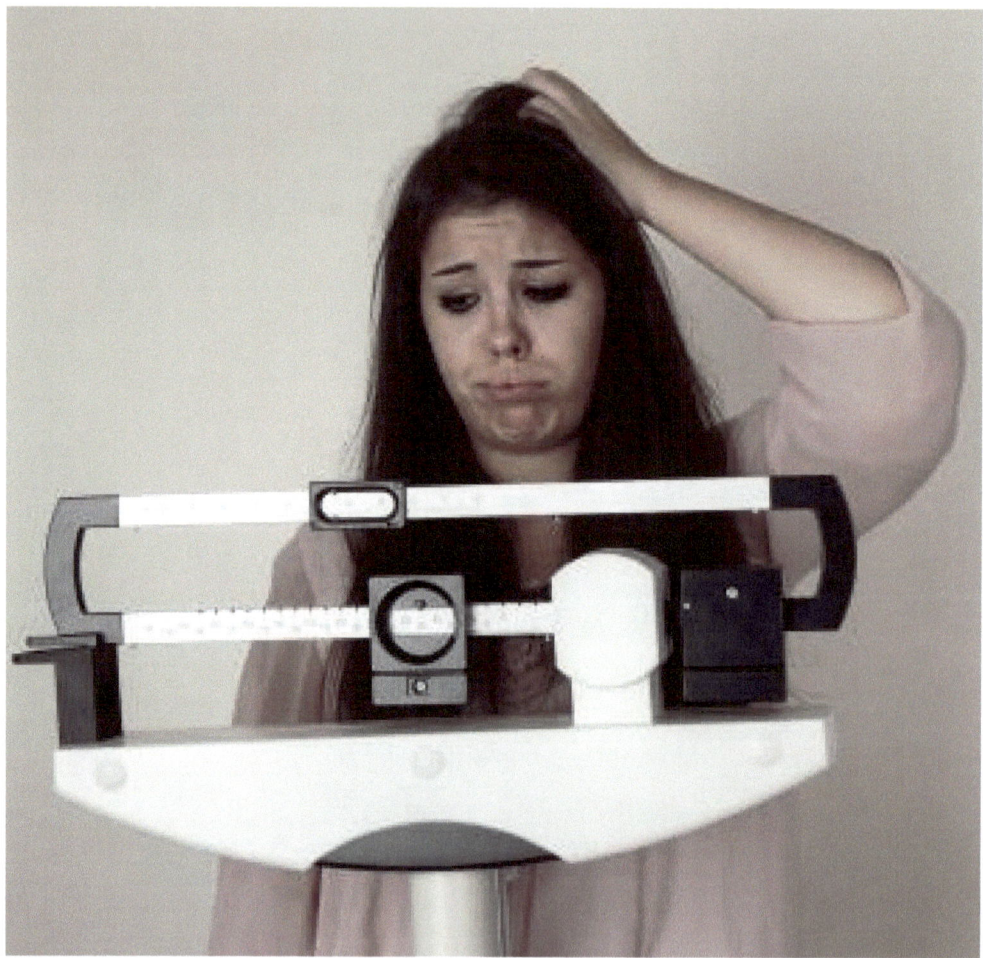

You can't control junk food cravings

Considering the facts, flour and sugar are one of the most addictive ingredients. This clearly explains what happens with fat people, and how they are not really responsible for their figures. In his book *Salt, Sugar and Fat*, Michael Moss tells the inside story; how junk food is actually made from such ingredients so that you get addicted to it. Sugar and flour are deliberately added into foods so that they can easily takeover your hormones, brain chemistry, metabolism and taste buds. Hence, it is perfectly normal to not being able to control your cravings for sugars and carbohydrates. Sugar is in fact now termed as the new nicotine, as it is almost 8 times more addictive than cocaine. This is the reason your willpower cannot win against your addiction. Detoxification gives you scientifically proven methods so that you can easily refrain from these types of hyper-palatable and hyper-processed foods or substances.

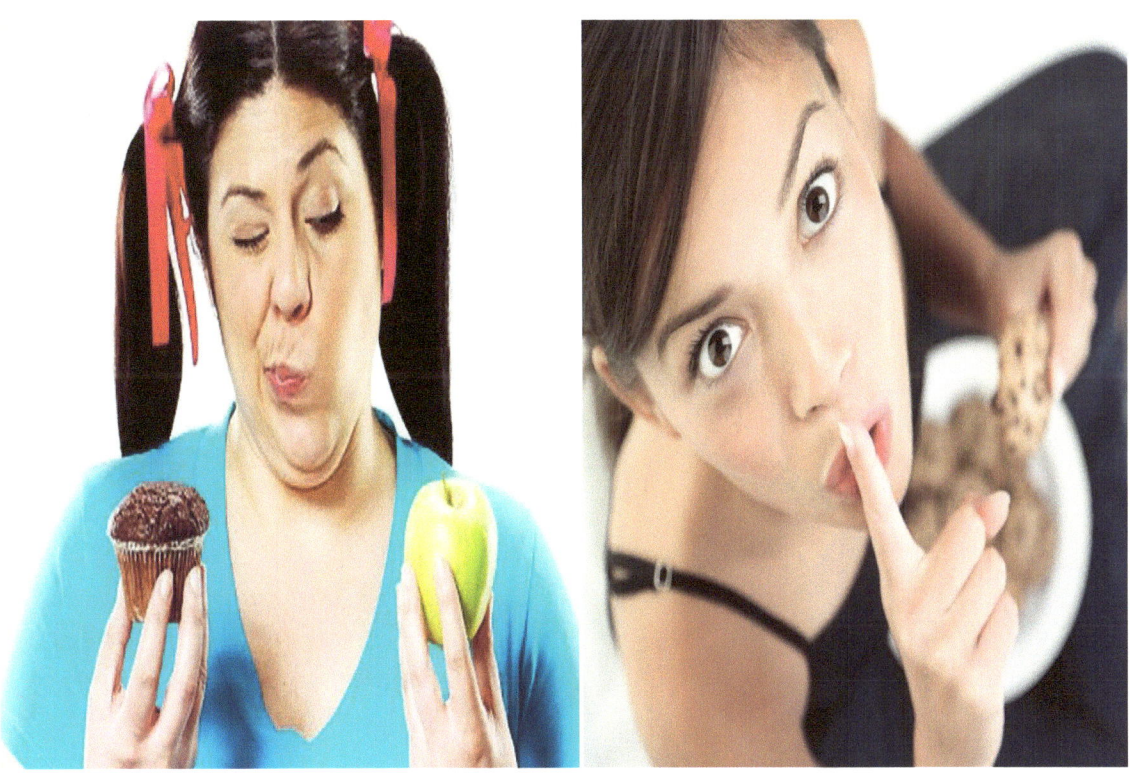

Giving time to yourself

The busyness and responsibilities in our lives have forced almost all of us to ignore ourselves completely. We all have chosen such eating and living habits that our bodies have become unhealthy, even if it's not so apparent. Too little exercise, junk food, too much stress and too little sleep are all those habits and lifestyles that contribute to our unhealthy selves. In these five days of detoxification program you can set free your body from toxins like processed foods, alcohol, sugar, caffeine and flour. Additionally, these five days are for you to simply work on yourself and nurture your body. Getting 7-8 hours sleep every night, deep breathing and healthy exercises all take you to a healthy mind and body.

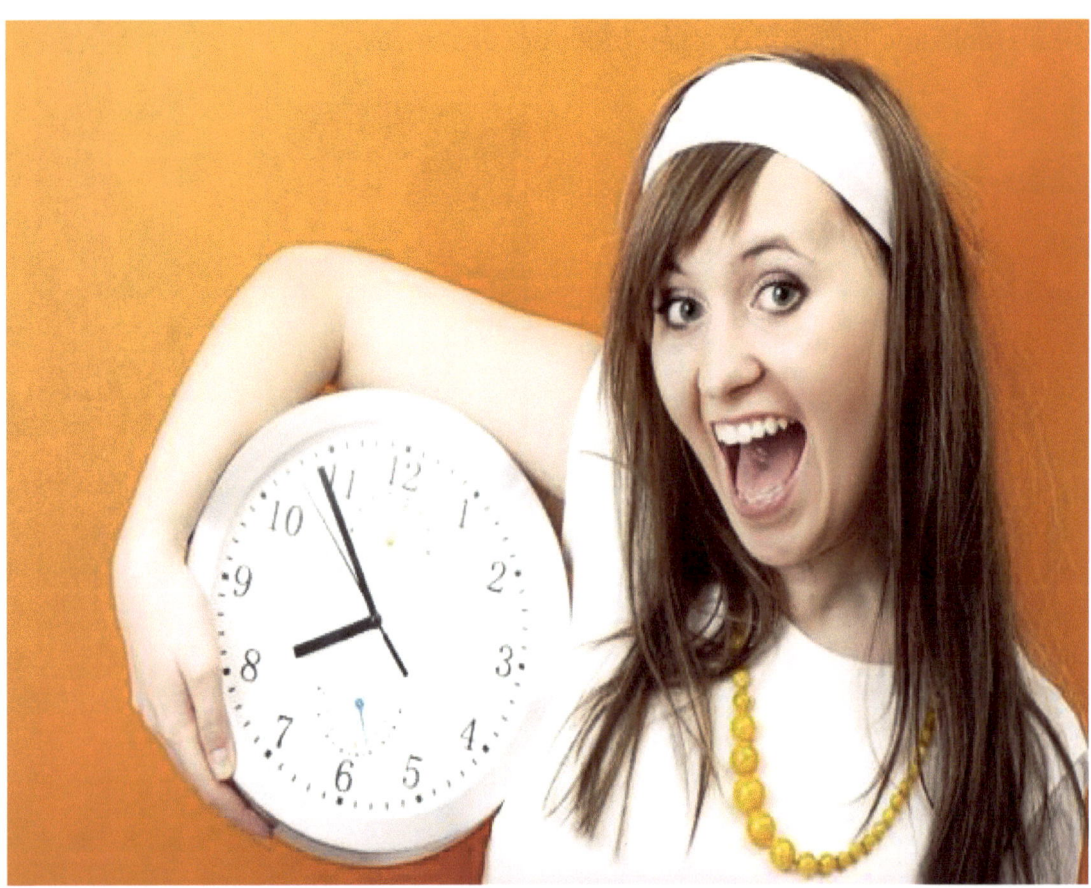

Never tried it before

As discussed earlier, it is extremely difficult for you to understand when your body needs you to control your diet. This is the reason that most of us have never tried to limit our diets to only fluids for a few days. You might seem to be completely normal but maybe your body has more potential. Detoxification therefore, is the quickest and the easiest way to recharge your health.

Better Breath

According to scientific researches, it has been concluded that backed up colon is one of the reasons of bad breath. Your body needs to get rid of these toxins, and for this reason most of the detox programs include colon cleanse. You will feel your breath improving once the toxins are removed and your digestive system starts to function properly again. However it is important for you to remember that your breath may get worse during the detoxification process; but you need not to worry, as it is natural for breath to worsen while the toxins are released from the body. After these five days, your breath will become more subtle, refined and better.

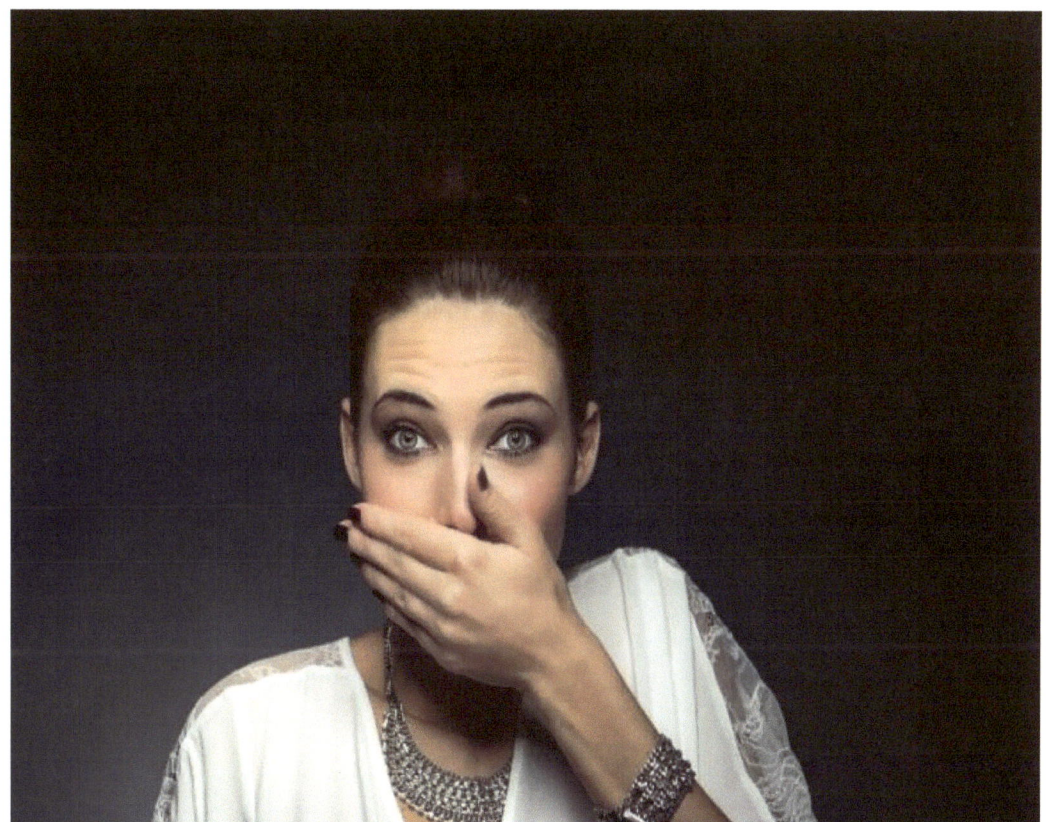

Better Thinking

Good detoxification programs always consider the working of your mind during the cleansing. During the time of cleansing and purging of toxins, it is usually advised to meditate so you can get in touch with your mind and body and both of them get more peaceful. Most people who have detoxed at least once in their lives accept that they felt their minds being very clear, and the feeling of fogginess faded away. Their claims are very much justified considering the fact the junk foods containing sugars and fats make our bodies lethargic and affect the ability to think and focus.

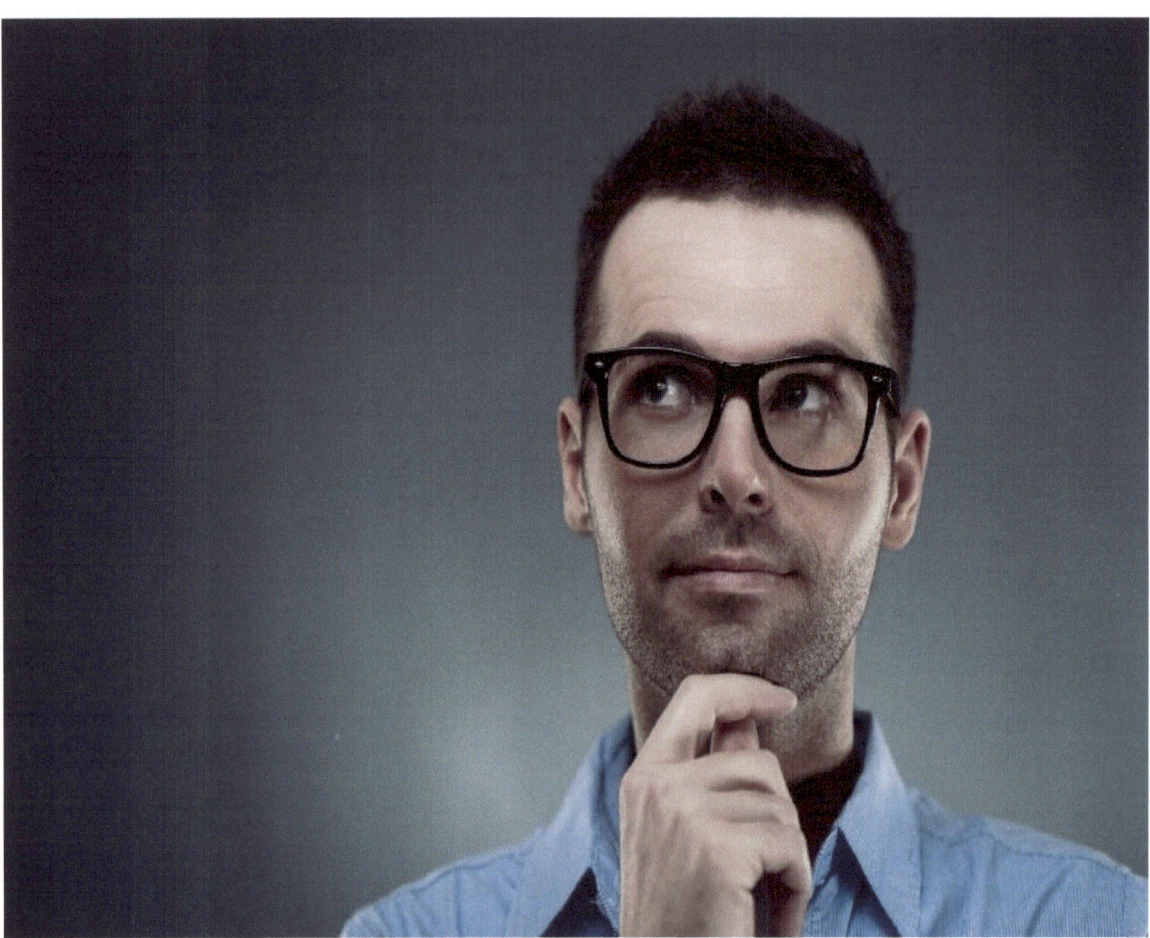

Healthier Hair

The growth of your hair occurs in the hair follicle. This is why by the time you realize something is wrong with your hair, it's already dead. This is similar to the functioning of liver; you never find out when it needs help. This is the reason it is important for you to take an action before your hair lose all their health and shine. As discussed earlier, detoxification is important to make your body keep working at its maximum potential. During and after the detoxification program your hair will be able to grow without any participation of the toxins that were there earlier in your body. This growth is definitely going to be very different from what you might have experienced before; your hair will now become softer and a lot shinier. In case of male baldness, detoxification will not be a complete solution. However, a quicker growth has been witnessed after detoxification, which is a sign of better health of hair.

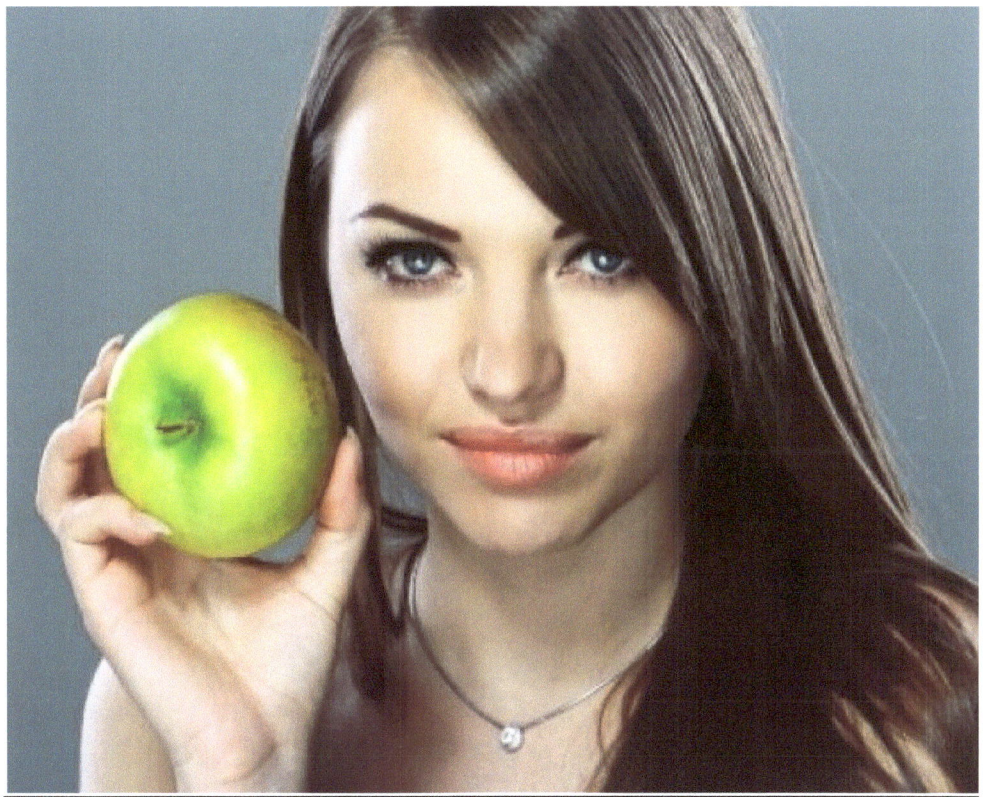

Anti-Aging Benefits

Almost everyone these days wants to look young and is worried about aging symptoms in a young age. What we don't know is that the constantly growing amount of toxins in our body is one big contributor of the aging process. One of the best anti-aging processes is detoxification as it reduces the damage faced by your body by releasing or transforming these toxins. By following the process, you will see both, short-term and long-term benefits. It is however important to note that you must not switch to the lifestyle which caused you to go for detoxification program. You must improve some of your living and eating habits permanently.

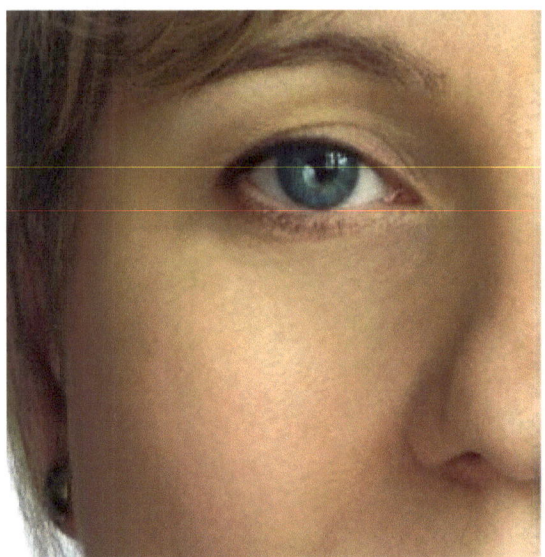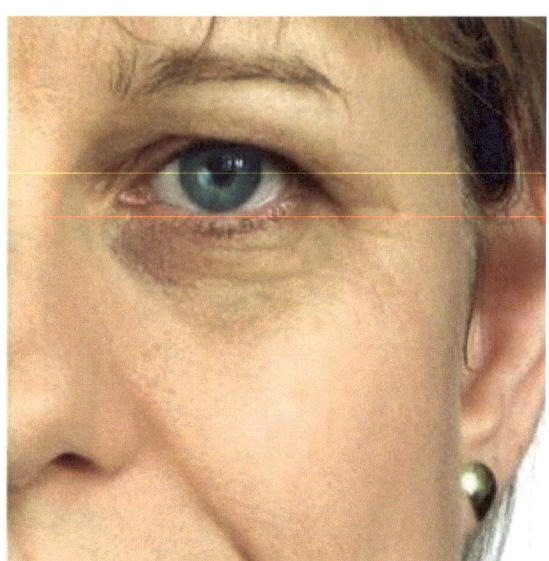

Wellbeing

As your health improves, you start feeling better. Hence we can say that detoxification generates a sense of wellbeing. Even though the programs are usually taken to lose weight or to improve overall diet, the best benefit of detoxification is the good feeling that you get. Feeling good also means that you will see improvement in all other aspects. Increased productivity, better relationships, good focus, all of this will help

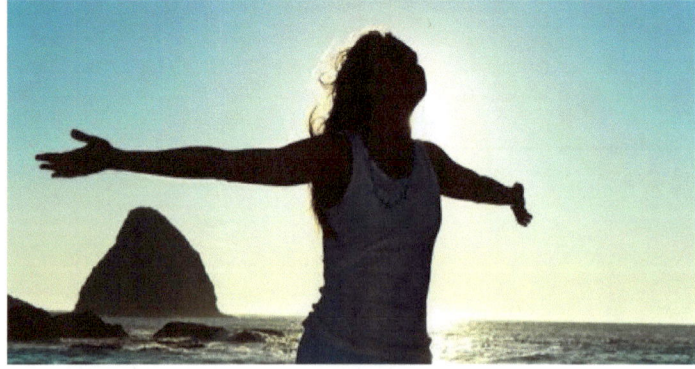

bring back zeal and energy in your life.

Improved Skin

As you might be already aware, skin is the biggest organ on your body; and this explains why your skin may benefit the most from this 5-day program. Some programs also advise to take a sauna, so that your body sweats out extra toxins. Some people have also reported that detoxification has helped them with acne. For others, the process helped them get a clearer, softer and smoother skin. Again, it is important to note that the condition of acne or the skin generally is likely to get worse during the process as toxins are being released. This is normal and in fact, it is to be taken as a green signal to show that you're moving towards betterment. During the detoxification process, there may be some signs of skin degeneration but do not worry because in the long term, your skin will generally improve greatly. The reason the skin faces side effects during detoxification are because it adapts to a certain toxin environment and inhibits it. However, once the process is complete, your skin will look clearer and much better than it was before the detoxification process.

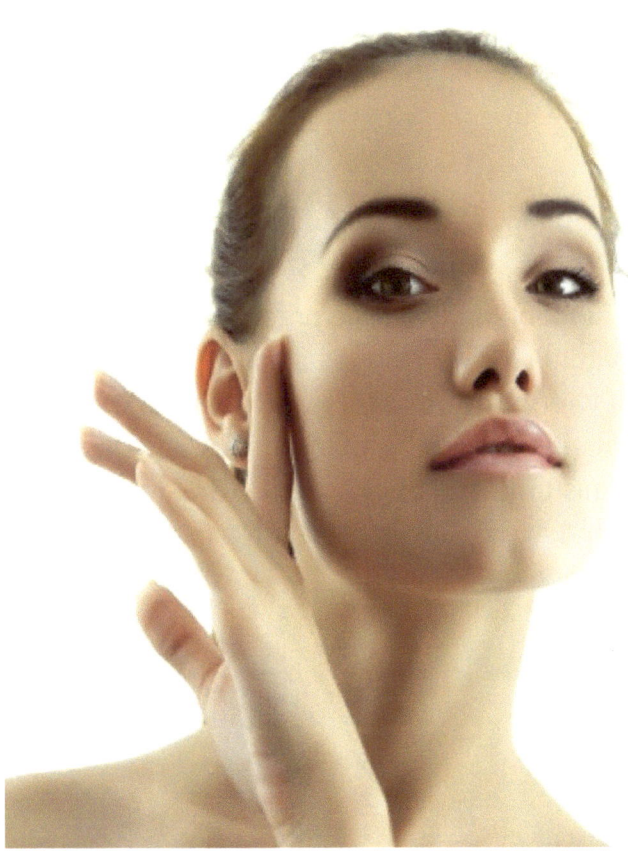

Losing Weight

As we know the change in diet during detox programs, we can easily understand how it causes a decrease in weight. Though, there is more to it; in the long term the whole process can help you change your unhealthy habits. The rapid loss of weight and reduction in calories is what is mostly advertised. It is true that detoxification reduces the calories and fats in the body rapidly, but at the same time it is equally important to retain the eating habits or else these changes won't stay. You will have to replace addictive junk foods with the healthier ones, and make regular exercise a habit in order to make your body stay as fit as it will be right after the process.

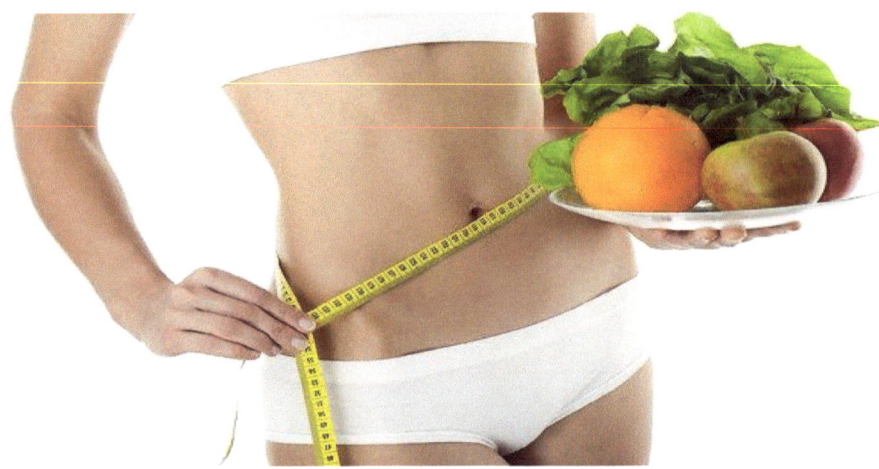

Stronger Immune System

Detoxification means optimum functioning of all the organs. This means that your body will absorb more nutrients like vitamin C, which boosts up the immune system to a great extent. The lymphatic system of your body benefits greatly from the herbs and substances you take in during the process, which helps in making you healthy and strong internally. The exercises during this time and after that also, help the lymph fluid to circulate throughout your body and excrete unwanted substances, which makes your immune system stronger in the process.

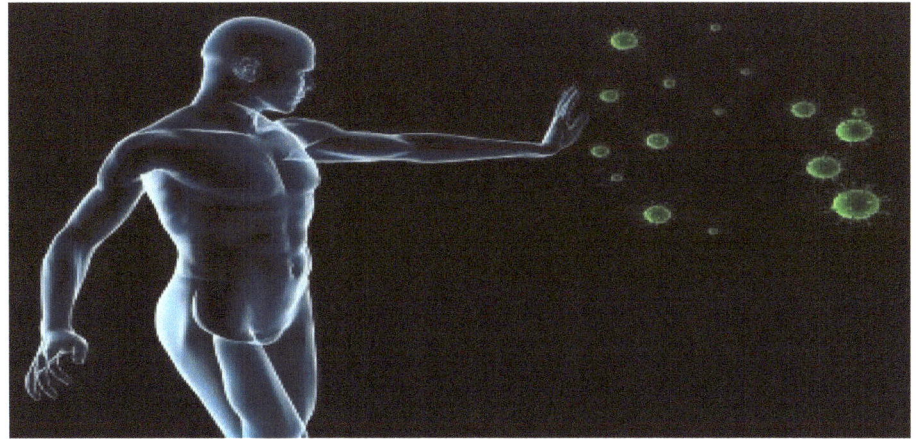

FRUITS, VEGETABLES AND COLORS

As discussed earlier, adding fruits and vegetables to the diet is one of the best ways to boost all your systems and your overall health. Each fruit or vegetable has its own composition of proteins and vitamins that are extremely important for your body. You might not even have to eat anything else if you take sufficient amounts of these fruits and vegetables. If taken regularly in the pure form, they definitely result in better health.

The main reason of adding them in your diet is to avoid eating animal products and other fats. Dairy products usually contain hormones and antibiotics that are earlier fed to animals. Cutting down these harmful products from your diet means avoiding high acid-load on your body.

However, people usually confuse detoxification with sticking to green fruits or vegetables only. Nutrition expert Dr John Berardi says, "The vibrant colors of fruit and vegetables tell us which disease-fighting nutrients they contain."

Purple:

Most Purple fruits and vegetables have large amounts of resveratrol. This helps in prevention of insulin resistance, a cause of diabetes. Examples include red wine, beetroot and blueberries.

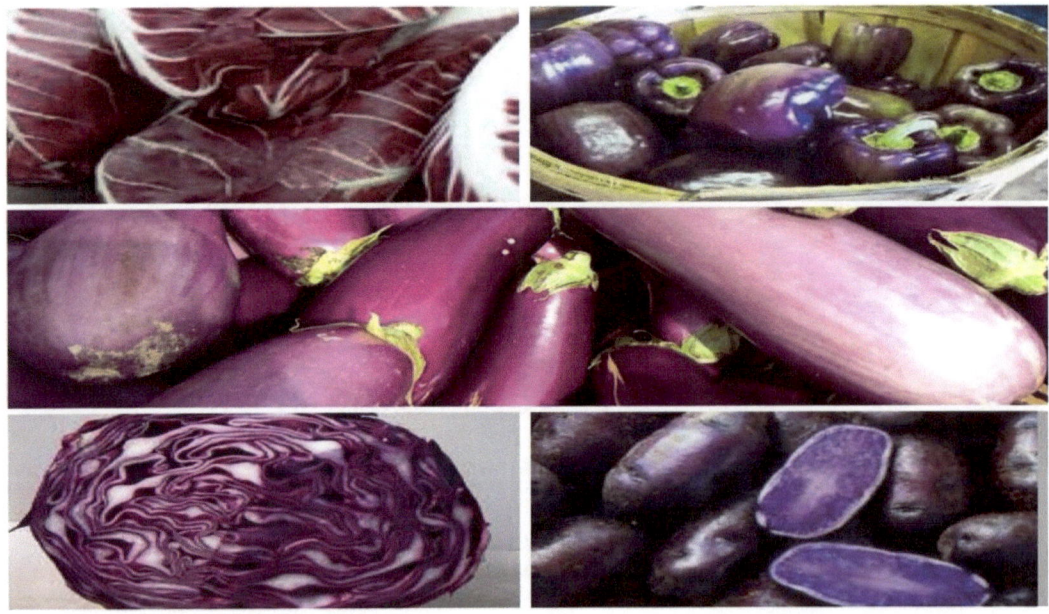

Green:

Green vegetables are mostly known for in flavonoids. These in flavonoids protect the cells in your body from damages, and also have anti-inflammatory benefits. Broccoli, spinach and kale are some of the most popular green vegetables.

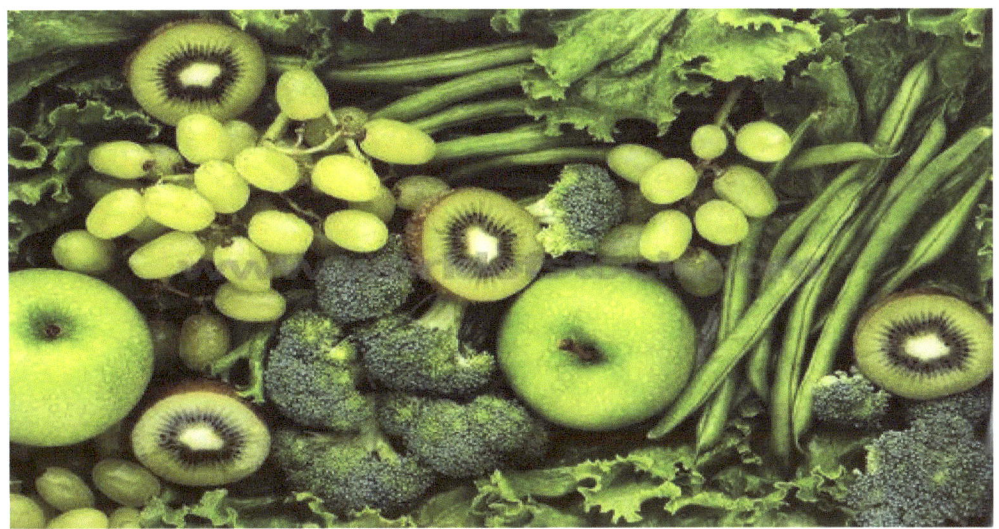

Orange:

Orange vegetables and fruits are mostly rich in beta-carotene. The body converts this beta-carotene into Vitamin A. This helps in keeping the eyes and skin healthy. Mangoes, sweet potatoes and carrots are some of the most common examples.

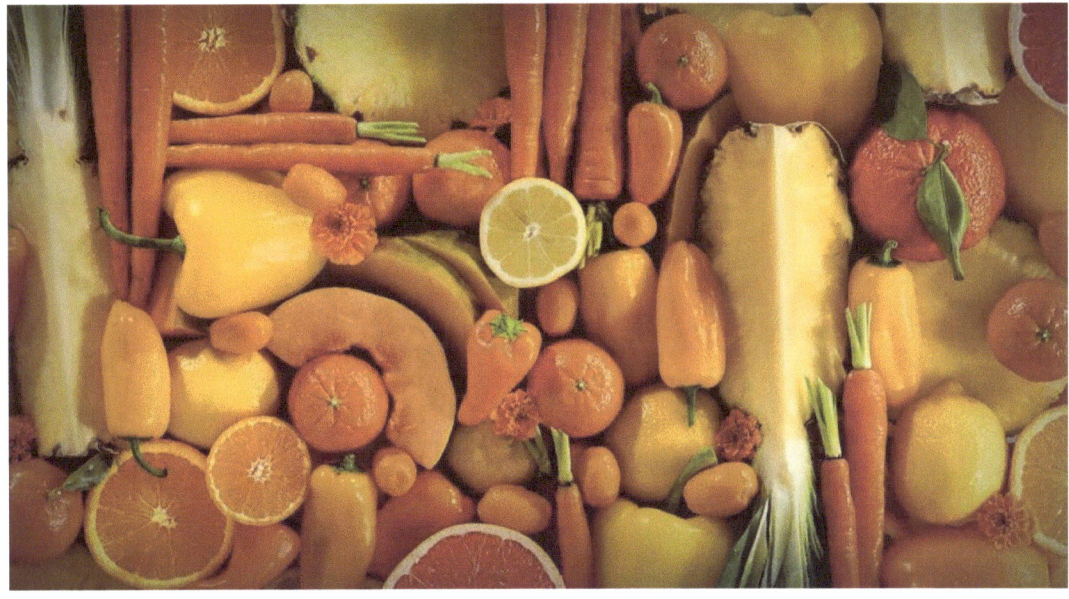

White:

White vegetables and fruits are all rich in Quercetin. This natural bioflavonoid is very helpful for skin, nerves, bones, sinuses, and most importantly, removal of toxins from the intestines. Examples are coconut, cauliflower and garlic.

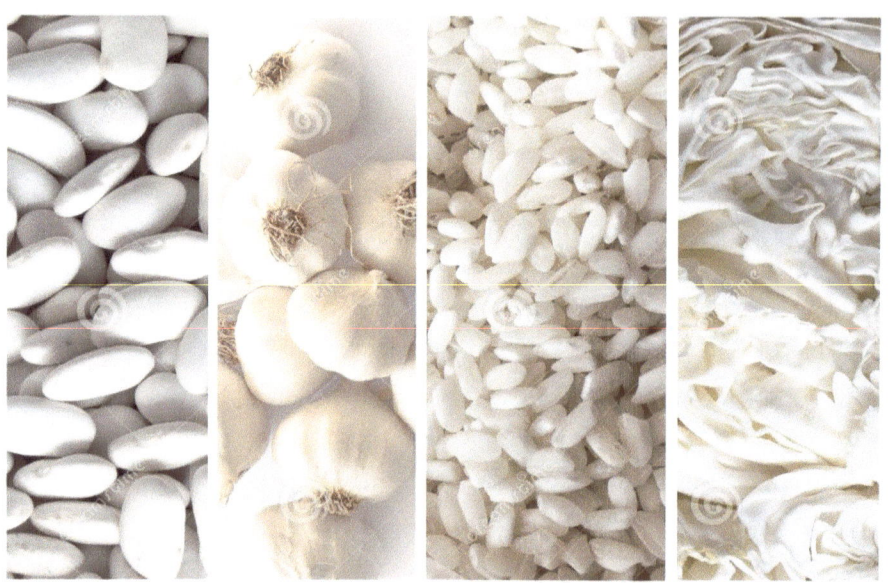

Red:

Red vegetables and fruits have lycopene. A study in Cambridge University concluded that lycopene is important for good functioning of blood vessels and minimizing the risk of cardiovascular diseases. Chilli powder, tomatoes and cherries are examples.

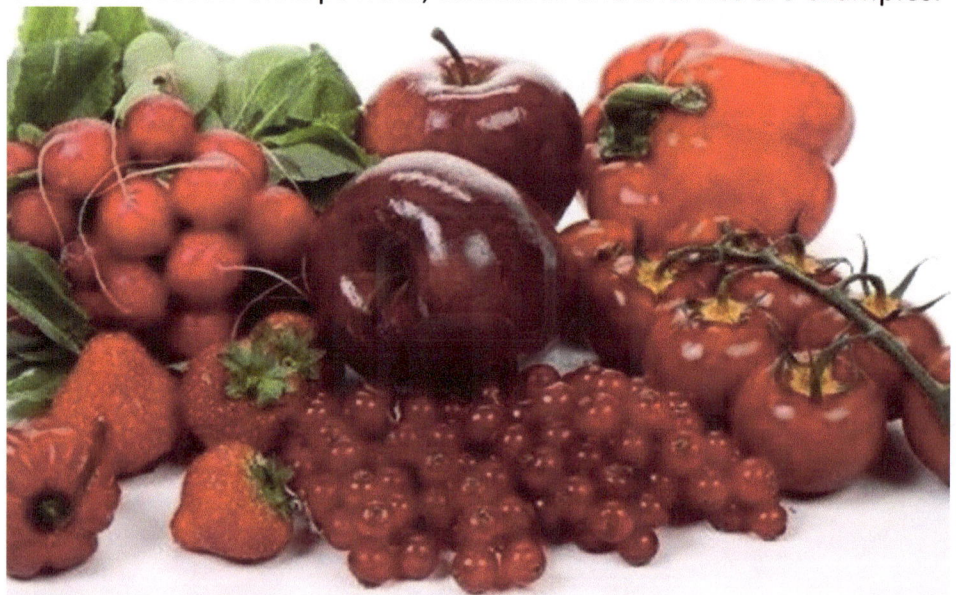

Regular Yoga:

There are numerous benefits of doing yoga regularly. It is essential to perform it for 20 to 60 minutes regularly. The art of yoga is not a difficult one to learn. You can always look up to find the most beneficial methods.

Drinking Lemon Water:

Water is said to be the most important fluid that your body needs. Making a habit to drink warm water with ½ lemon juice first thing in the morning can make your body a lot healthier than before.

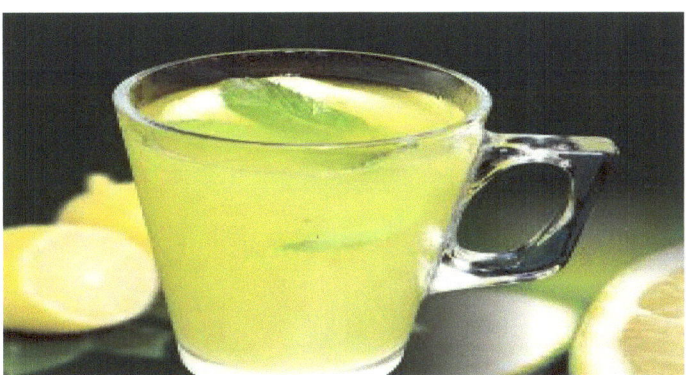

Drinking lots and lots of water:

Other than the lemon water, drinking just water is another very important tip. The amount of water your body needs depends on your age and the weight of your body. It is recommended to drink ounces of water equal to half of the ounces of your body weight daily.

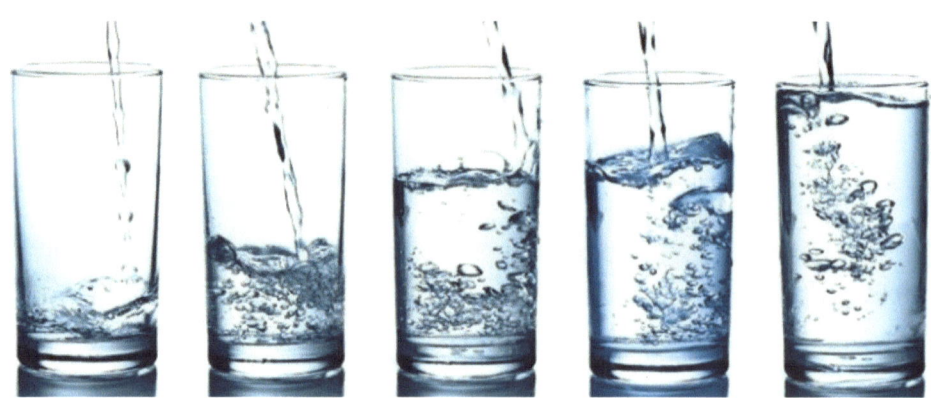

Dry Brushing:

We discussed in the previous section the role lymphatic system plays in making our immune system stronger. Dry brushing is one method to stimulate this system. You should scrub your body with a dry brush before you take shower. This will remove dead skin and help in releasing toxins from your body.

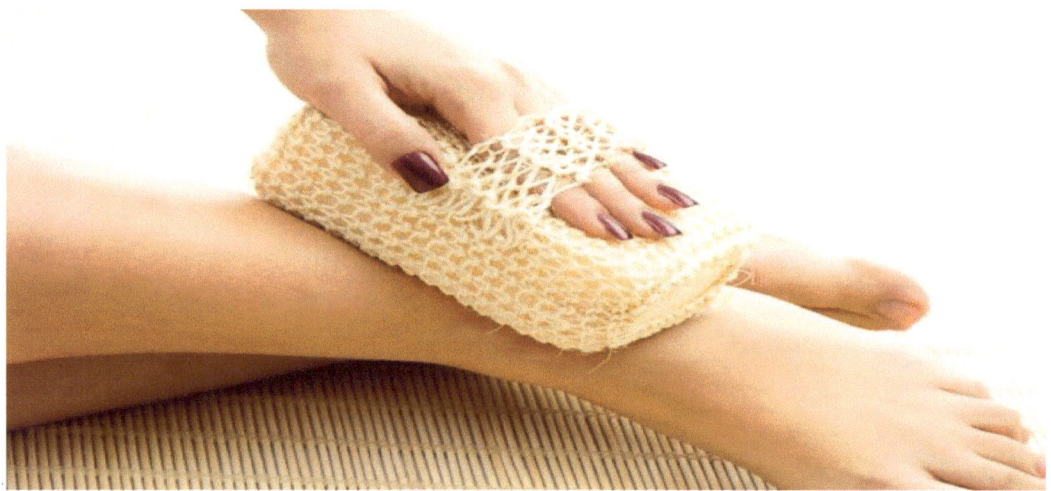

Take in Magnesium:

Most people have a deficiency of magnesium in their bodies that can be there due to various reasons. In any case, to counter magnesium deficiency, it is imperative that you take a magnesium supplement at night before sleeping. It will help you to sleep properly for the rest of the night, which is an important part of the detoxification process.

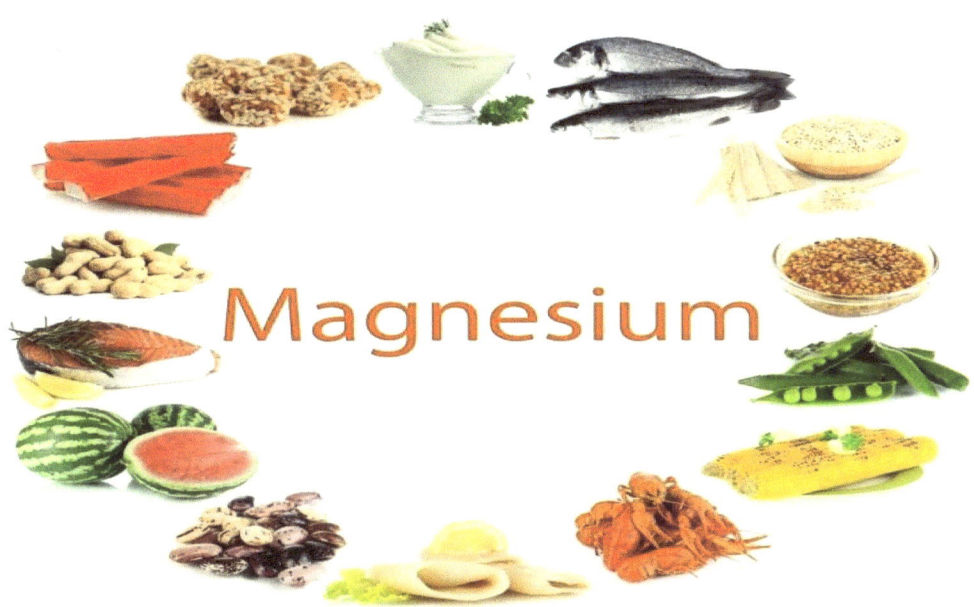

Sweating:

This is one of the most triggering factors when comes to detoxification. The type of exercise is your choice, but sweating is important to detox the body by releasing additional toxins.

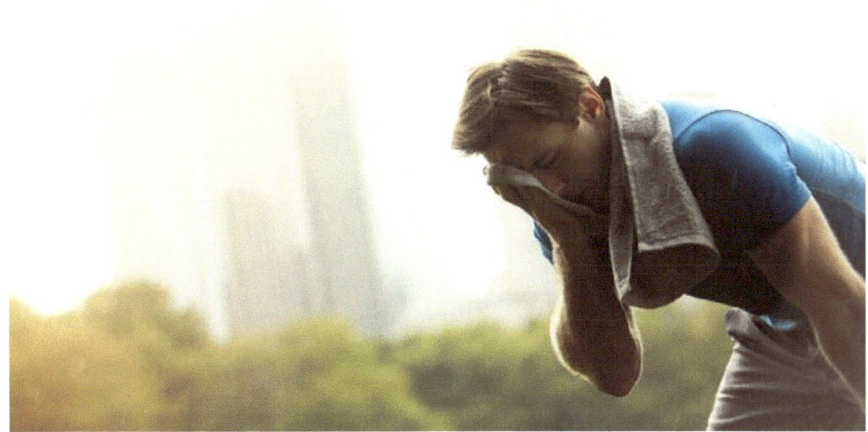

Resting:

It is one of the ignored components of the detox process. Getting enough rest during the day is as important as getting enough sleep at night. This is important because during the process your body can be exhausted and fatigued, which is likely to make you get irritated before you experience being all healthy and happy. Your body needs to know that what it's facing in these five days is just temporary, and feeling great is not very far.

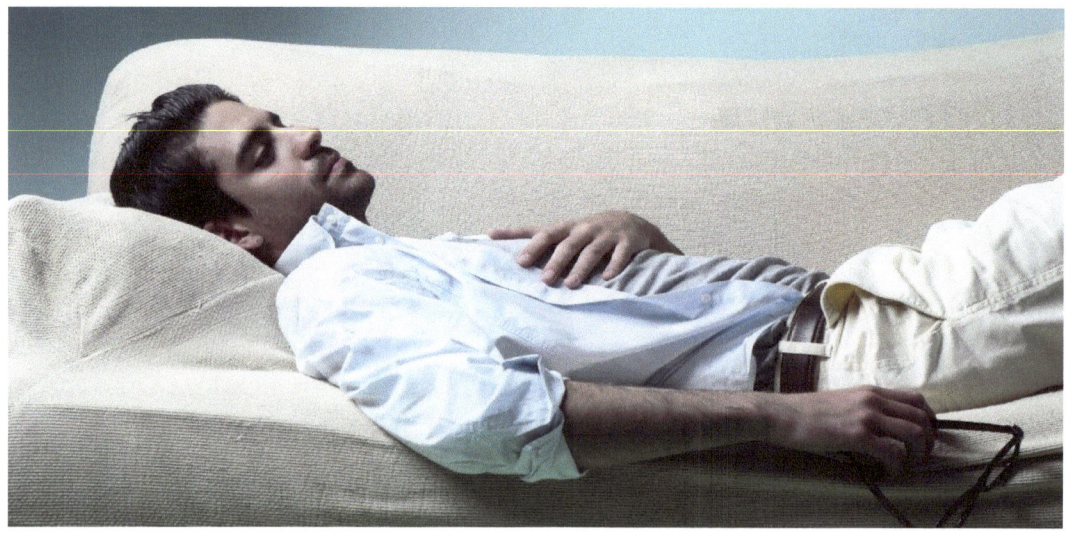

CARBOHYDRATES: SLOW BURNING, NOT LOW QUANTITIES

Slow burning carbohydrates (carbs) help nourish your body by providing your digestive system with the right balance of minerals. They help boost your metabolism and enable you to be healthier and more energetic. These slow burning carbs are rich in fiber and minerals and help you in controlling and reducing the effects of various types of diseases. This section discusses the various types of carbs that can be a part of your diet and the benefits of each type of carb along with the extent to which they should be a part of your diet.

Eat freely with Green Carbs!

- Low glycemic load (GI) vegetables are very beneficial for the health. These green carbs benefit your body in numerous ways and help you fight various diseases. Fill your plate with greens that include broccoli, lettuce, asparagus, cauliflower, Brussels sprouts, cucumbers and many others. They help you grow and nourish your body leading to better health and increased energy.

- Minerals such as iodine, calcium and iron are essential for the body and help boost metabolism. Important and rich sources of these minerals are seaweeds. Sea vegetables are tasty and can help add flavor to your dishes. They greatly benefit your digestive system since they help restore balance to the body by decreasing acidity, acting as a detoxification agent. They are also quite helpful for improving digestion and breaking down certain foods that include beans.

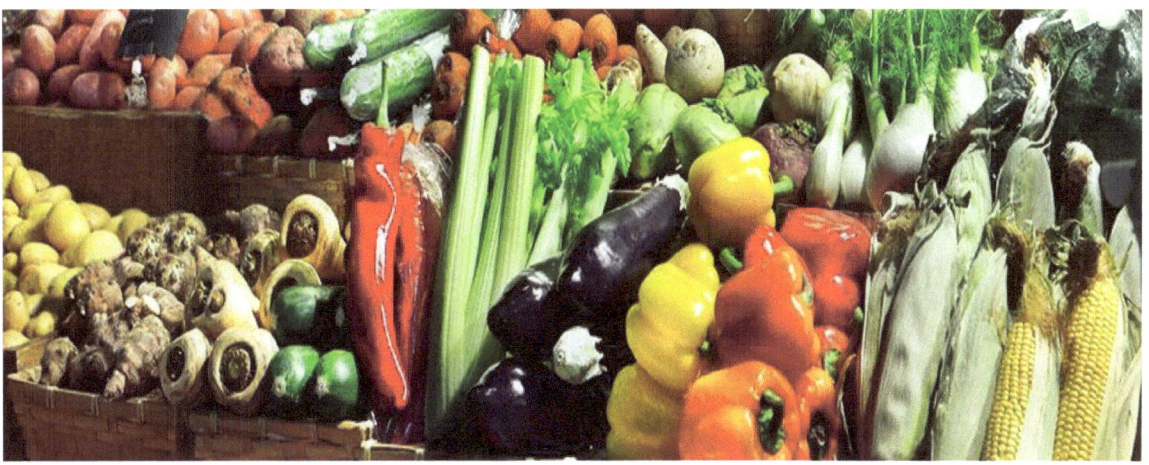

Consume modest amount of Yellow Carbs:

- Grains are yet another type of foods that have low GI. They provide necessary nutrition to your body. However, not all grains are slow burning; this needs to be kept in mind. Whole grain cereals, pastas and various other grains are not considered to be slow carbs. The following, however, are slow burning yellow carbs that *should* be a part of your diet, but only moderately: Quinoa, amaranth, buckwheat, brown rice, black rice, tortillas, whole wheat bread, rolled oats and teff.

- Beans and Legumes are a rich source of protein. They are healthy carbs that digest slowly and provide sustained energy to the body. Some beans are also full of minerals that include zinc and iron. A few options you can consider as part of your diet include kidney beans, black beans, pinto beans, adzuki beans and black-eyed peas.

- Fruits are always beneficial to the body, particularly fruits that are slow burning. These fruits that include nectarines, plums, peaches, apricots and apples can add to your diet and be a delightful to eat yet helpful to the body. These fruits can benefit the body by reducing cholesterol and blood sugar and hence help in fighting a number of different diseases

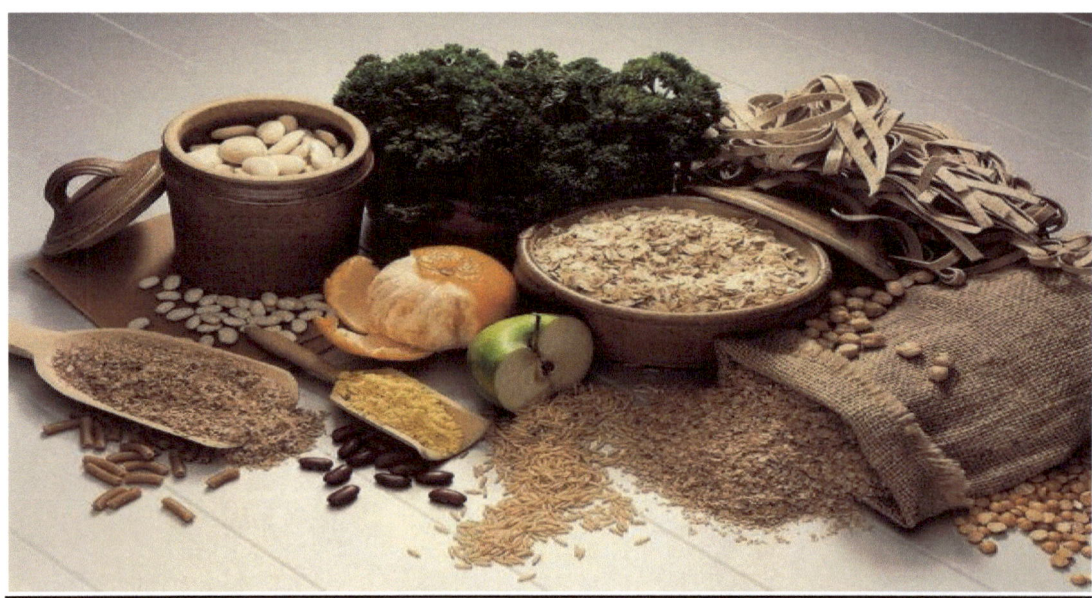

Page 36

Red Carbs – Just a few:

- Red carbs have the highest GI among all types of slow burning carbs. It is very important to keep a check on how much of your diet consists of these. Though they are helpful in the body, they tend to be more quickly digestible than the rest of the slow burning carbs. They are rich in nutrition and should be a part of your diet but only a limited amount. Some examples of red carbs are sweet potato, yam, pumpkin, parsnip, winter squash, grapes, bananas and fruits that are packed with juice (such as oranges).

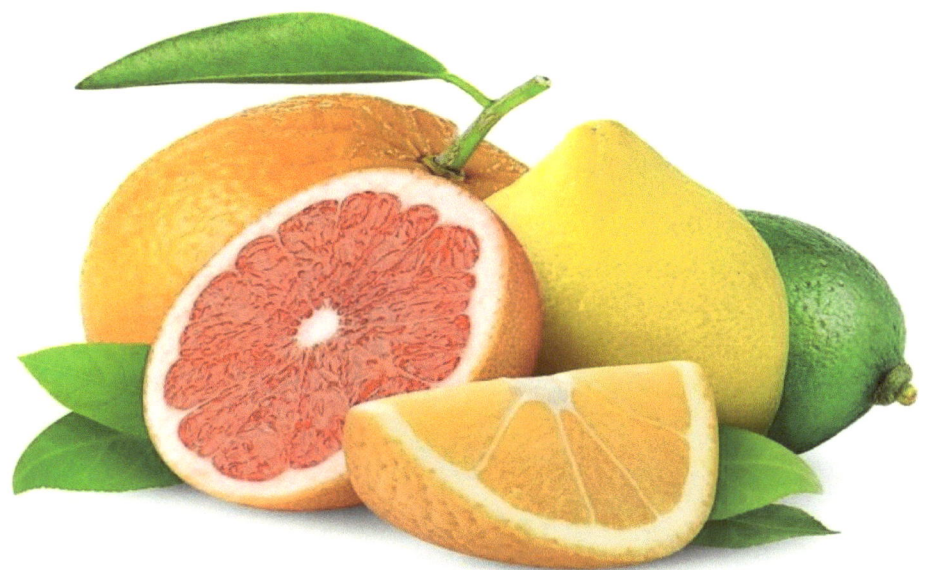

Carbs you need to avoid:

Here is a list of carbs that have a high glycemic load and hence can be the cause for different types of cardiovascular and digestive diseases. These should be completely avoided in any form. These forbidden carbs include:

• Resistant Starch.

• Whole Grains (including barley, einkorn, spelt, wheat, cereal).

• Dried Fruits (such as raisins, walnuts).

• Processed carbohydrates since the minerals and nutrition in the carbs are stripped from these.

NUTRIENTS IN YOUR PLANT BASED DIET

A vegan diet is a well-balanced diet that helps benefit the body in a number of ways. However, when sustaining a vegan diet, the importance of nutrients needs to be considered as well. Although a vegan diet is known to be well balanced and nutritious, it is not completely true. The reason is the lack of a proper meal planning in most diets that leads to insufficient consumption of various nutrients that include calcium, vitamin B-12, omega-3 fatty acids, iron, vitamin D and high quality proteins. This section highlights the importance of each of these nutrients and how you can fulfill your body's need for these nutrients by making subtle additions to your vegan diet.

<u>Calcium</u> –The myth is that the use of dairy products is necessary to fulfill the daily calcium requirements. The truth, however, is that you do not need dairy products in your diet for these nutrients. Calcium is a vital nutrient for the bones and they help you develop stronger and healthier bones. Considering your vegan diet, you can add dark leafy green vegetables (such as cabbage, collards, mustard greens), broccoli, Brussels sprouts, fortified soy and fortified tofu to your diet to help nourish your body with sufficient calcium intake.

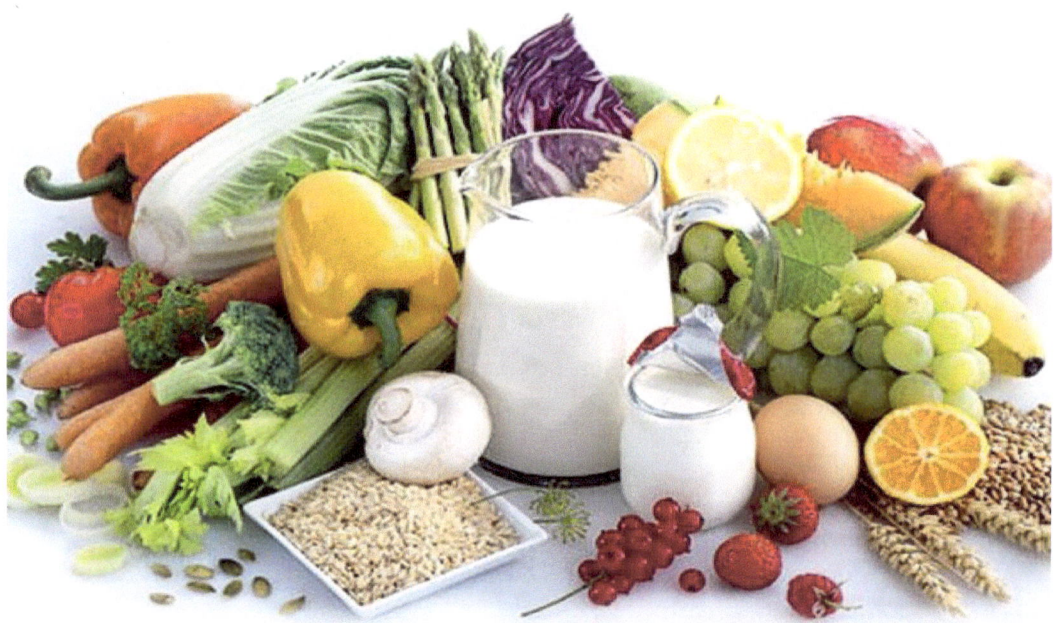

<u>Vitamin B-12</u>- These are nutrients that are mostly found in animal products and hence, it can be difficult for a vegan to fulfill the daily requirements of this vitamin. However, these can be accounted for in your daily routine by adding *substantial* amounts of soy and rice milk beverages to your diet. Apart from these, if you prefer an ovo-vegetarian then the consumption of omega-3 eggs can also help with supplying your body with these nutrients since these are known to be rich in Vitamin B-12.

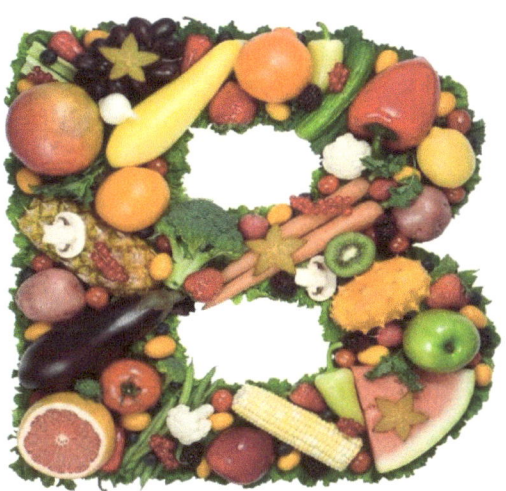

<u>Omega-3 Fatty Acids</u>– Omega-3 fatty acids help the digestive process in your system by producing enzymes that help in breaking down food for use by the body. This regulates the digestive system of your body. These can be found in a number of vegan diet products such as walnuts, flaxseed oil, soybeans, hemp seeds and chia seeds.

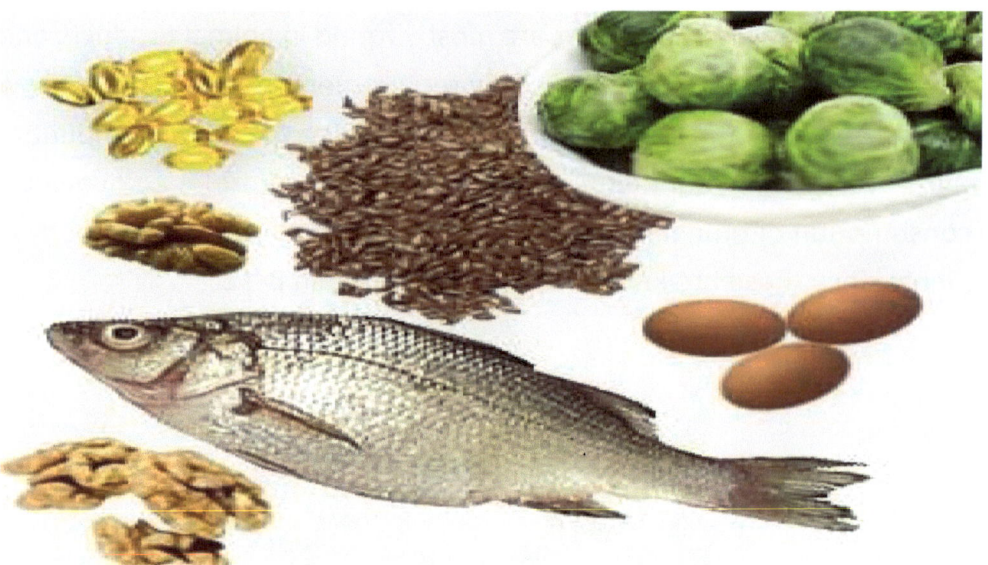

<u>Iron</u> – Iron is an important nutrient for the body. It is necessary for growth and the production of blood cells in the body. Iron is a nutrient that can help the body recover and stay healthy, it boosts metabolism and that enhances the body's ability to fight bacteria. Vegan diet has been known to be associated with iron deficiency and this is the problem with such a diet. This is because of the lack of a balanced diet. There exist a number of good sources that can be combined. Adding subtle amounts of these food products can nourish your body with the required daily amount of iron. Fortified tofu, cooked green vegetables, beans and lentils are good vegan sources of iron.

Another problem with the consumption of iron is that it is not readily absorbed by our bodies. To increase absorption and decrease the iron deficiency, the following should be followed:

- Combine good sources of Vitamin C with your iron-rich diet sources to increase absorption. These include berries, tomatoes, lemon and broccoli.
- Avoid caffeine in any form especially tea since this contains compounds that make iron harder and hence, more difficult to absorb.
- Calcium and iron are not a good mixture. High-calcium foods need to be avoided at least for half an hour before the consumption of iron-rich sources. This is because of the fact that calcium curbs the absorption of iron.
- Iron pots should be used for cooking (iron-rich sources especially). This is because the acid in the foods attracts the iron in the pots and hence the amount of iron in the foods increases (almost up to ten fold!).

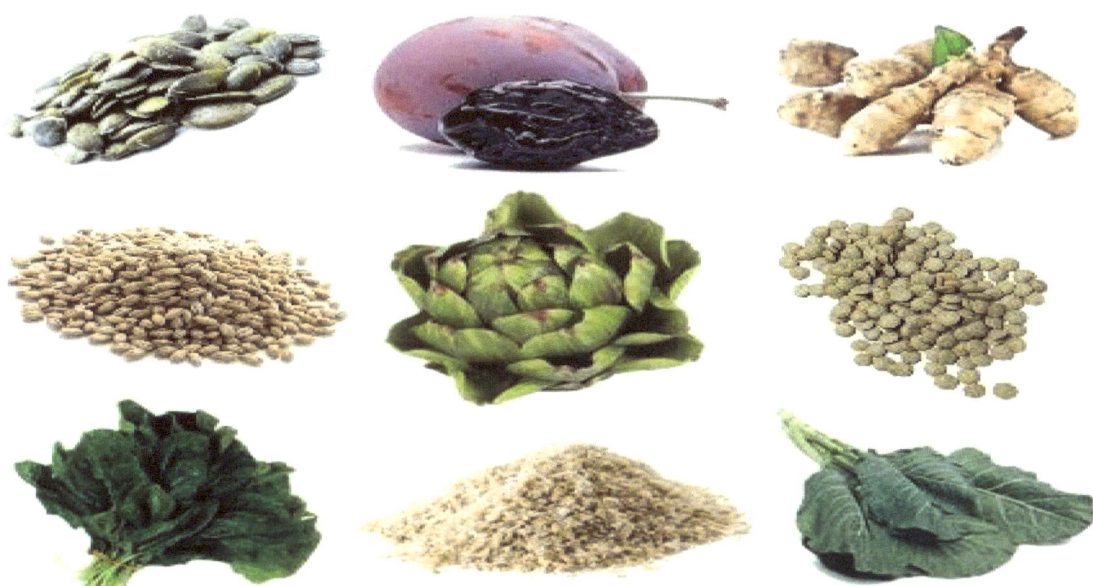

Proteins – These are nutrients that are absolutely vital for the body. Proteins are made up of amino acids that are obtained by breaking down the protein during the process of digestion. These amino acids produce glucose and hence provide energy to our system. They are also responsible for the growth of our muscles. Proteins is the fuel that 'drives' our body and enables it to work, hence they are the first and foremost requirement by the body during starvation. This highlights how important proteins are for our body. Here is a list of food sources that are rich in proteins and need to be a part of your diet:

- **Beans and Legumes:** Chickpeas, lentils, kidney beans.
- **Nuts and seeds:** Walnuts, Hemp seeds and Almonds.
- **Whole soy products:** Any products that are organic and non-GMO.
- **Whole food protein shakes:** Hemp, rice, pea or even high quality soy protein powder can be used to make protein shakes that can be consumed early in the morning for providing sufficient protein intake for most of your day.

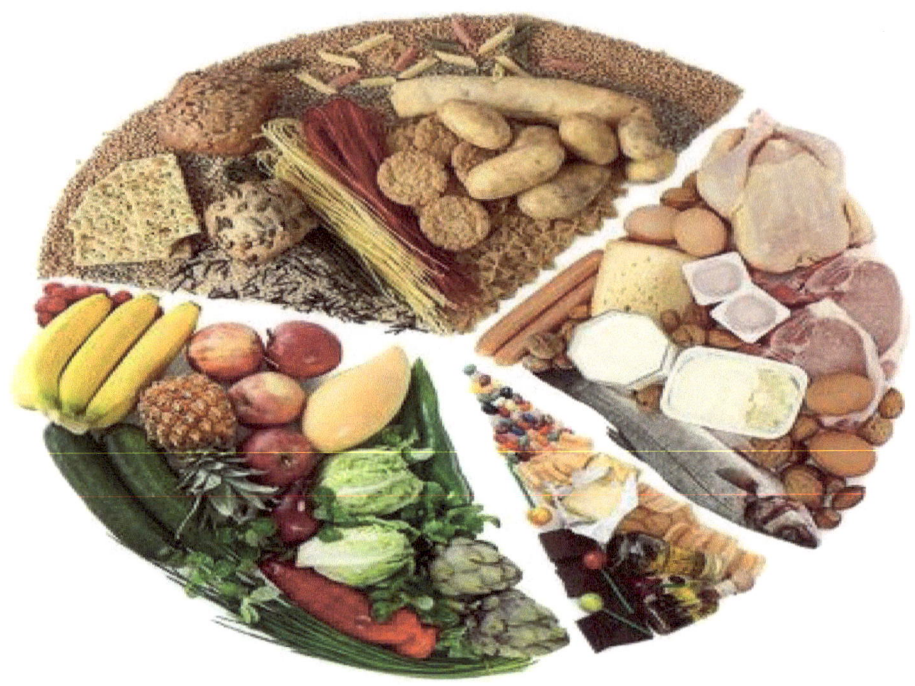

Vitamin D – The sun is considered as the prime source of Vitamin D. However, no matter how much your exposure to the sun, the amount of Vitamin D you absorb is never sufficient to fulfill your daily requirement. To ensure the consumption of Vitamin D and helping your body gain this necessary nutrition, it is important to take supplements for the Vitamin, irrelevant of dietary preference. Other sources of Vitamin D include fish, cereal and whole grains.

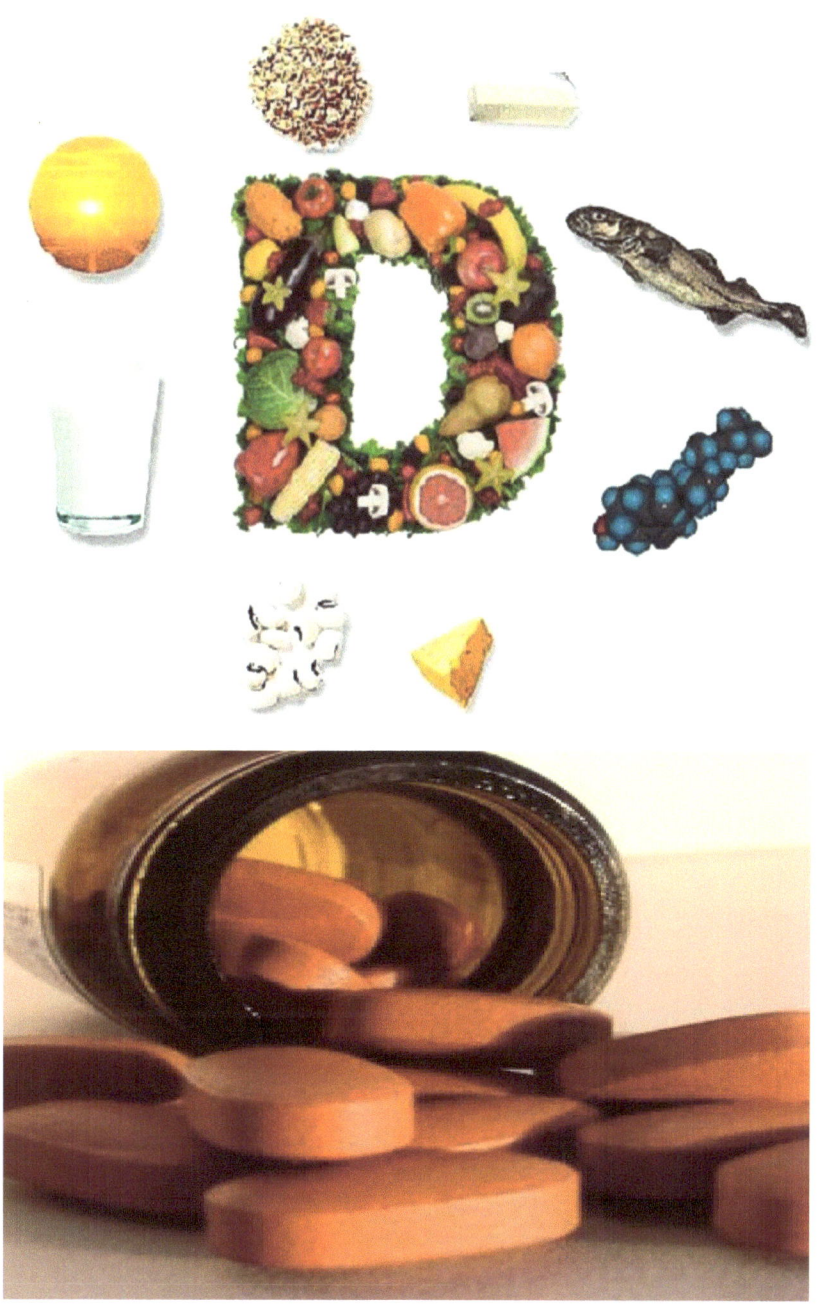

CHOOSING THE RIGHT FATS

Fats are not harmful to your body and they do not make you 'fat' on their own, this is a common belief among many and this is wrong. Fat, like carbohydrates and proteins are nutrients for the body and they are a necessary component that needs to be present in your diet. The reason is the vital role that fat plays for our bodies. The main feature of fat is that it provides us with energy, among the three micronutrients mentioned above, fat plays a major role providing the source of 'fuel' to our bodies and our brain. Apart from this, fats help our bodies maintain healthy skin, hair as well as body temperature.

We discussed the importance of fats in our bodies, now we shall discuss what actually needs to be a part of our diet and what doesn't. What you need to realize is that there are two types of fats, good fat and bad fat. Your aim is to ensure that you consume the good fat and avoid the bad fat and this can be done simply by taking care of your diet. Some tips on how to increase the intake of good fats that benefit your body are given below:

Change your oil: Avoid soy oil because it contains 'bad' fat that is not good for the body. Instead, you must use other oils that are available and will benefit your body such as walnut oil, virgin olive oil for use in salads and sesame, coconut, grape seed and sunflower oil for baking.

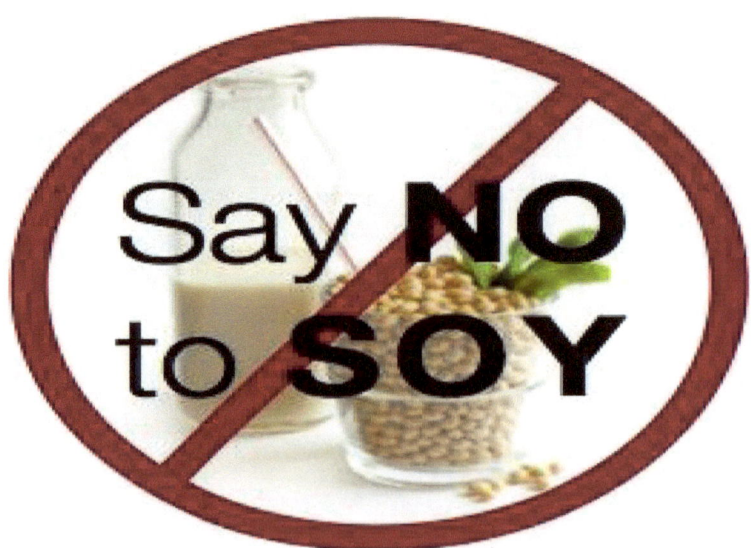

<u>Choose the right fats that are anti-inflammatory:</u> It is important to know which types of fats are beneficial to your body. The fats that are healthy and good for the body include:

- **Omega-3:** These are fats that help provide your body with sufficient nutrients and energy for sustenance. These include flax seed, borage, hemp and chia seeds. These can be added in minor quantities to your daily diet to provide the right amount of fat needed for your body.

- **Monounsaturated Fats:** These are smaller chain of fats and since they are unsaturated, they are more readily and easily used by our bodies. Sources include olives, avocados and olive oil.

- **Saturated Fats, healthy ones.** These exist too if you know what to eat. These are rich sources of fat but when taken in the right amounts they can help nourish your body. For instance, coconut butter is a rich source of Saturated Fats.

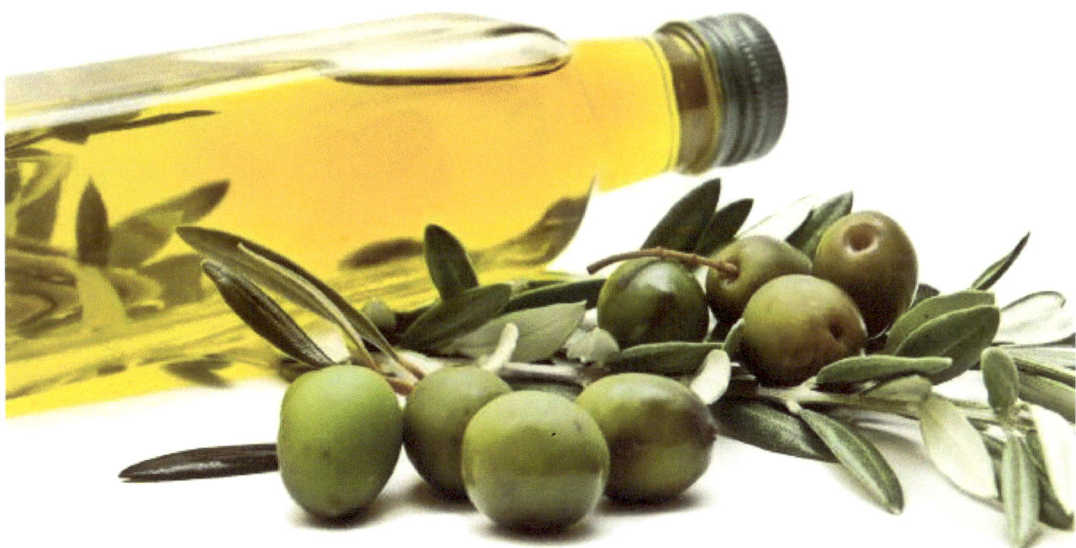

Page 45

FEW MOST IMPORTANT FRUITS AND VEGETABLES

ARTICHOKES

Artichokes help your liver function at its best, which eventually results in better removal of the unnecessary or harmful substances from your body. Artichokes basically increase the production of bile by the liver. Since bile is what helps in breaking down the foods we eat and using the nutrients in them, it is beneficial to increase the bile production.

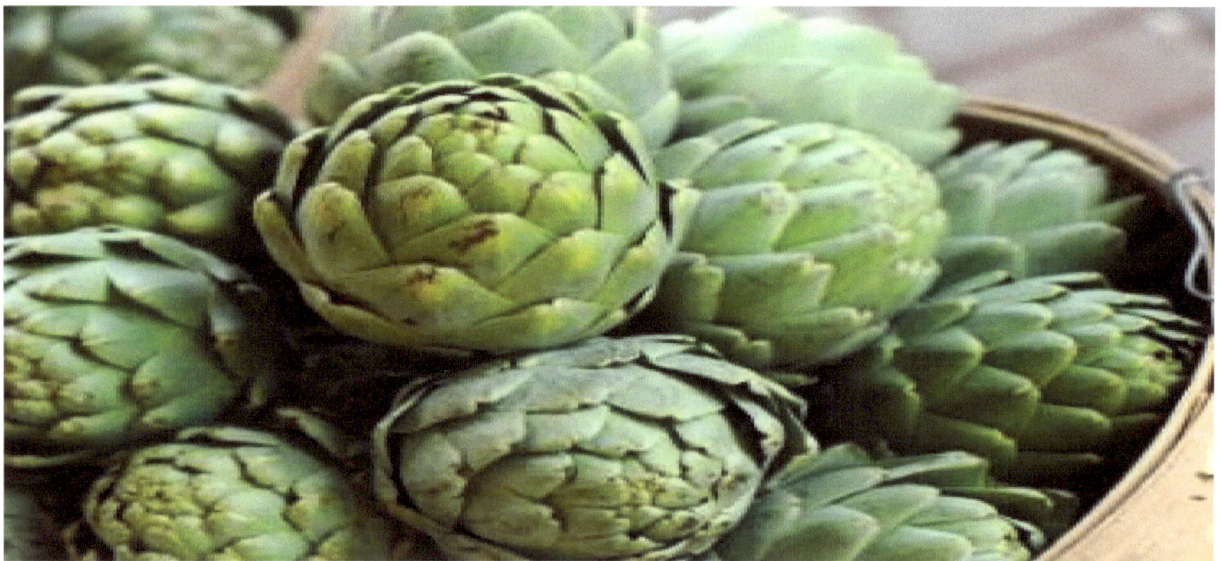

ALMONDS

Almonds are rich in Vitamin E. Just an ounce of almonds contains approximately 7.3 mg of vitamin E and that too in the form that body prefers. Almonds give you calcium, fiber, magnesium and protein which help in balancing blood sugar levels.

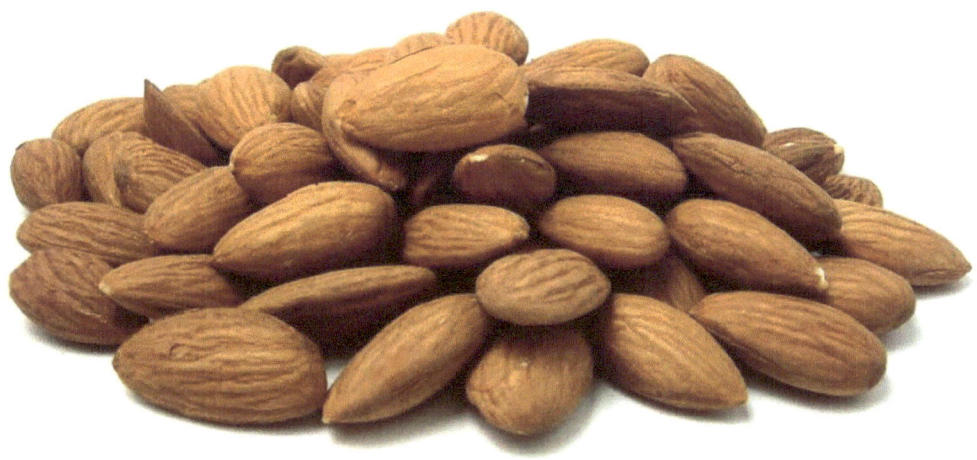

APPLES

Apples are very famous because of the nutrients they contain; vitamins, fiber, minerals, and all that the body needs. Apples also contain healthful phytochemicals like terpenoids, flavonoids and D-Glucarate. All of these play a very vital role in the detox process. Phlorizidin, a flavonoid is said to stimulate the production of bile, which helps liver in getting rid of toxins. Similarly, apples contain fiber pectin which is an important soluble for detoxification. It is often suggested that organic apples should be eaten as the non-organic ones have found to be amongst the foods that contain the most amount of pesticide residues and have 15% less antioxidant capacity.

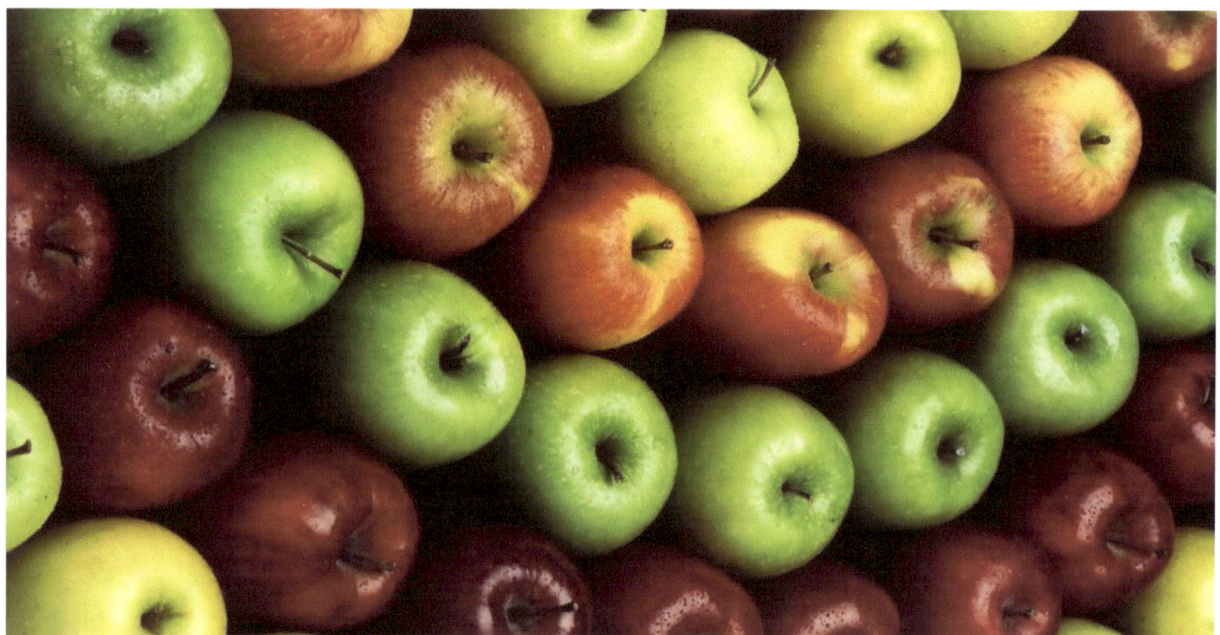

ASPARAGUS

Asparagus actually does a lot more than helping in the detox process; it keeps the heart healthy, gives protection against cancer, and gives anti-aging benefits. This anti-inflammatory food also helps with liver drainage. Additionally, it can reduce the risks of death from breast cancer and increases the chances of survival.

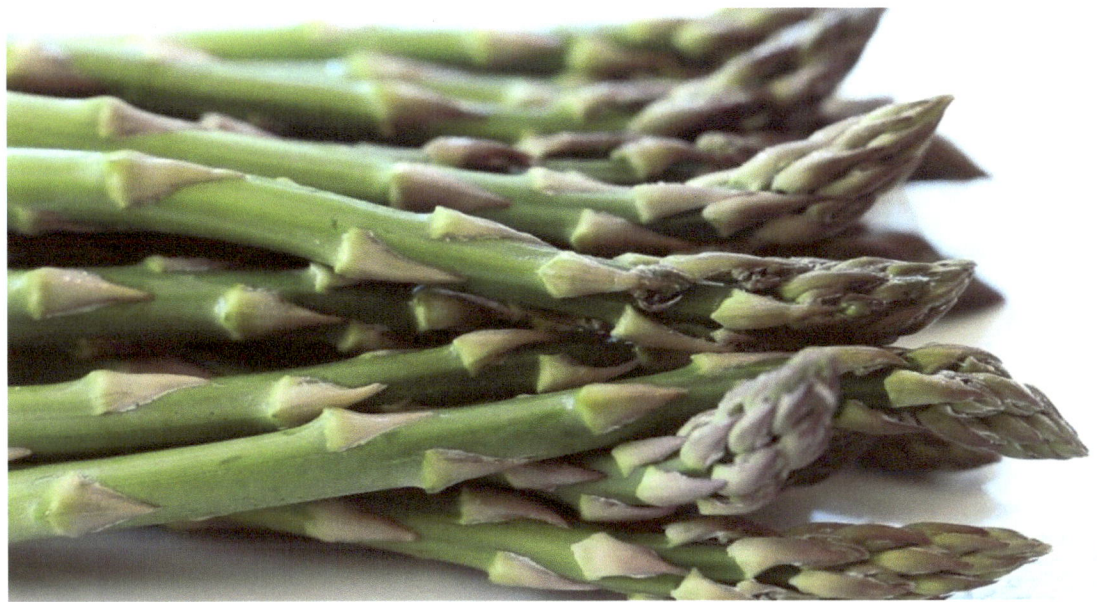

AVOCADOS

Avocados are full of antioxidants. They lower the cholesterol levels and block the toxins that destroy arteries. A nutrient named glutathione is avocados is capable of blocking at least 30 different carcinogens and help the liver in detoxifying synthetic chemicals. Glutathione is known to keep elderly people healthier and protect their bodies against arthritis. Lower metabolic syndrome risks, good diet quality, lower body weight, smaller waste and high good cholesterol are all results of eating avocados

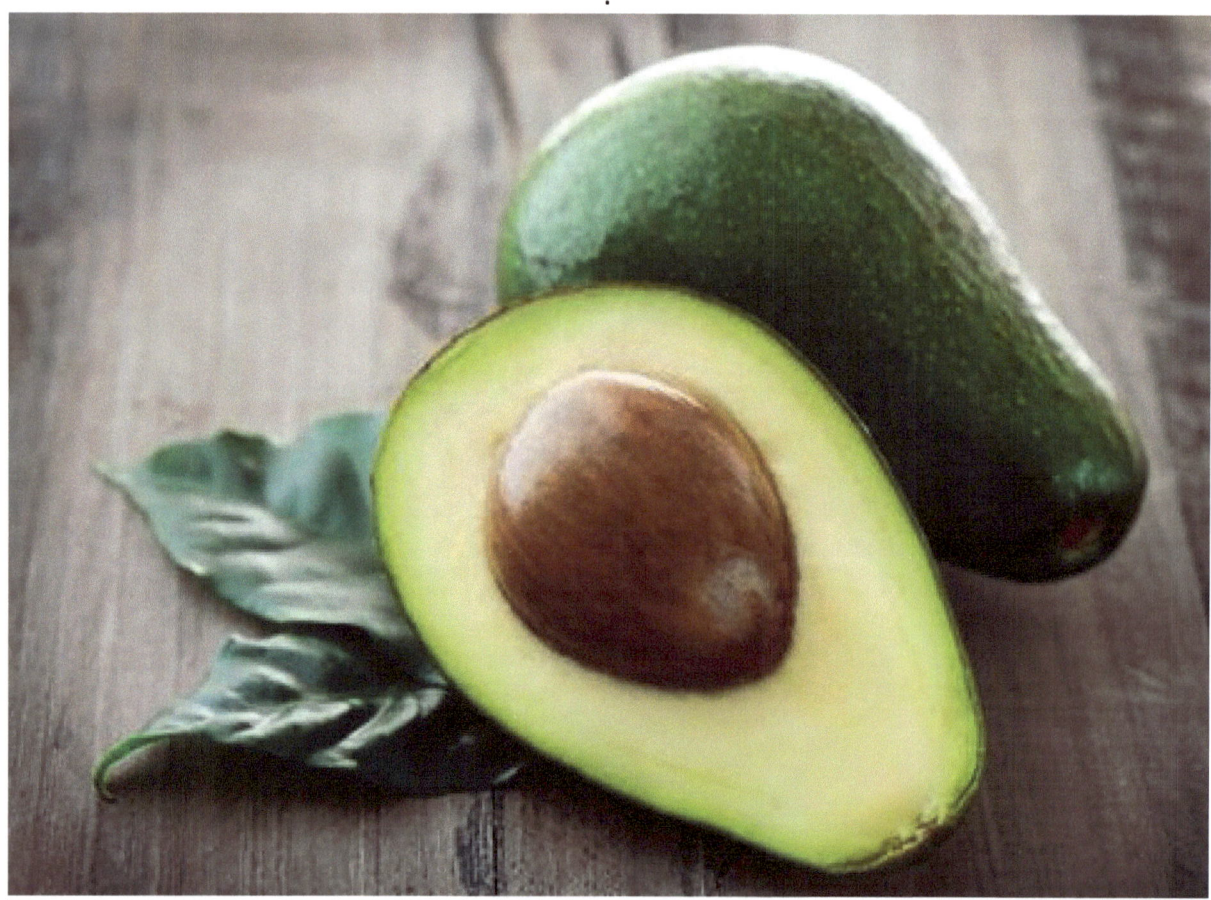

GRAPEFRUIT

Grapefruits are known to be wonder fruits because of their ability to detoxify, refresh and energize the body. Grapefruits are known to treat diseases and replace medicine without any side effects at all! This is the reason behind the popularity of the fruit. Not only this but they taste delicious as well, the juice-filled fruit can be consumed in a number of ways that include eating it as is after peeling off the outer layer. Grape fruits help treat diabetes, they prevent weight gain by eliminating belly fat; they lower cholesterol levels and even help with reducing gum diseases. Another particularly important known fact about grapefruits is their ability to fight cancer cells and help with cardiovascular problems by preventing a number of diseases and conditions. The nutrient filled fruit is delightful to eat and is a recommended addition to your diet.

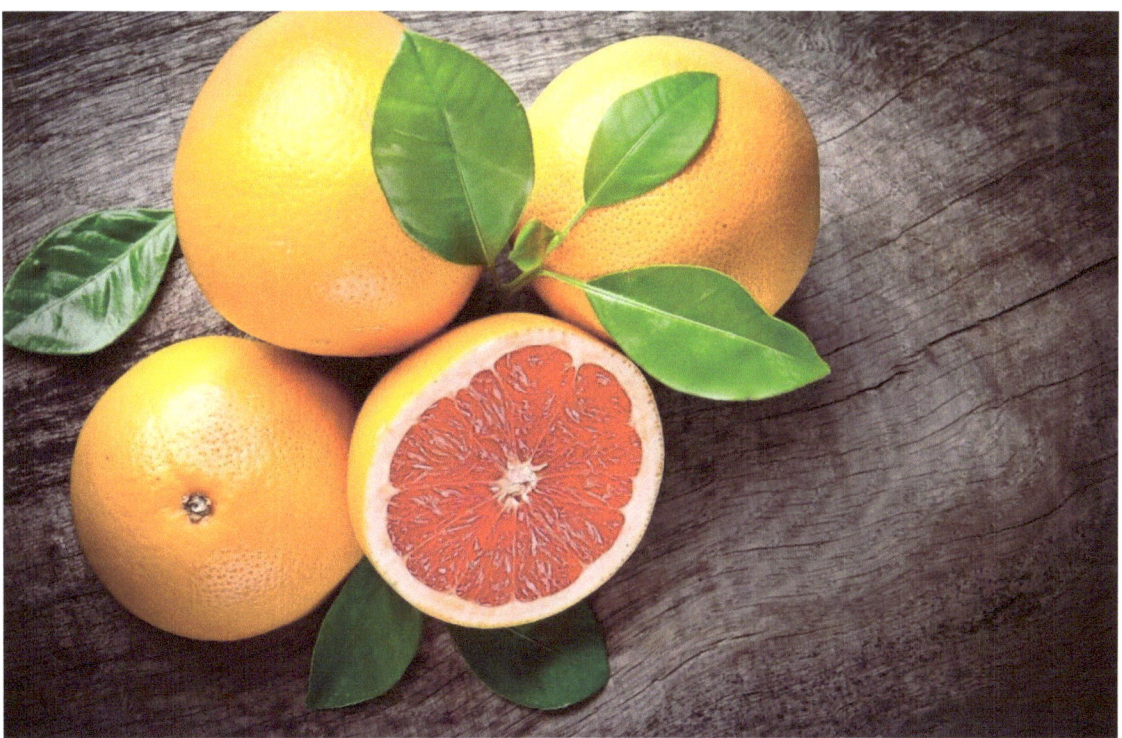

GREEN TEA

Green tea is a great addition to any form of diet and in particular, detoxification programs. The reason is the high level of antioxidants in green tea. It provides antioxidant polyphenols in large quantities with a catechin called epigallocatechin-3-gallate (EGCG). This is the reason behind the numerous health benefits of green tea. Discussing the benefits of green tea, it is particularly helpful in the detoxification process since it helps lower blood sugar, it helps remove toxins from the body and induce a healthier environment within our bodies to help it to develop and grow. Green tea is known also to enhance brain function by increasing neurotransmitters in the brain. It is also known to promote fat loss and lower the risk of developing cancer and various other diseases by boosting our immune system.

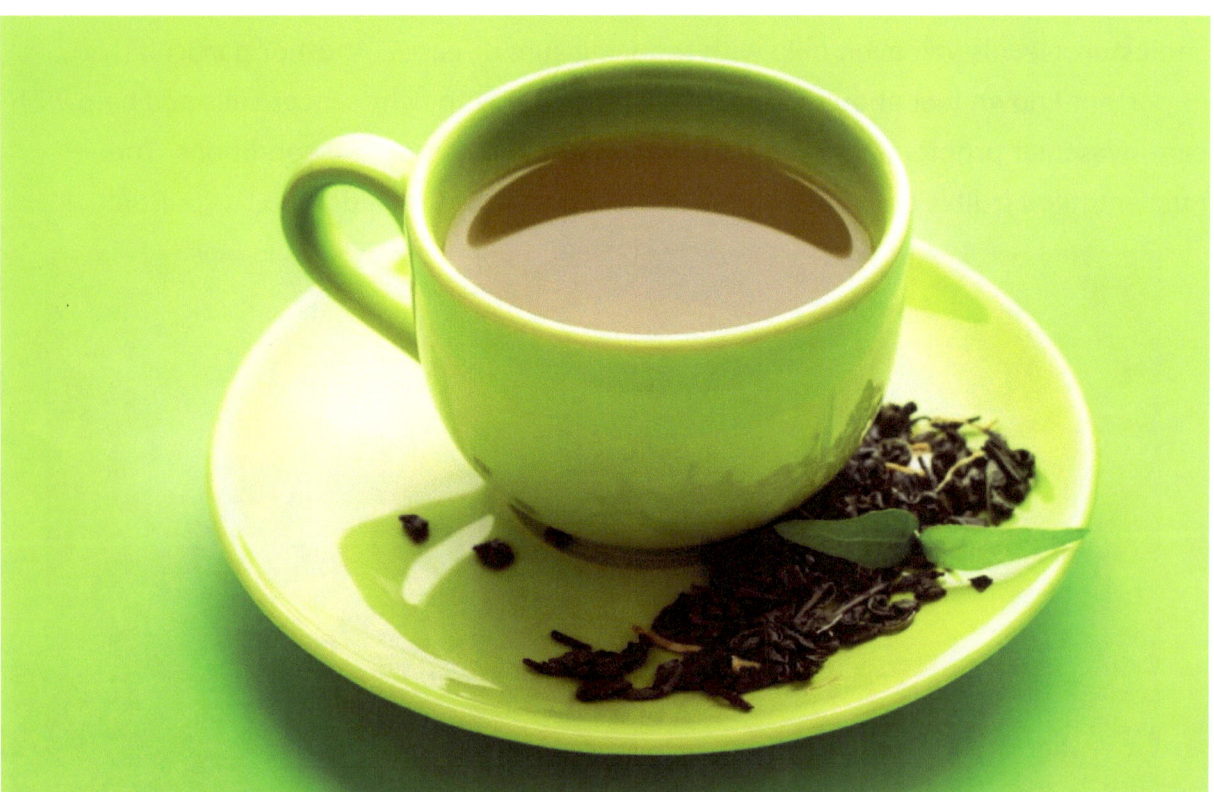

LEMONS

Lemons are stimulants that release enzymes to help with the chemical processes taking place in the body. Lemons are also known for their acidic nature and this helps in converting the toxins in the body to soluble form that ensures that they can leave the body through excretion more easily. Lemons are also a rich source of Vitamin C that is an essential nutrient for the body. Lemon water is an alkali that helps with several processes in the stomach and liver. They help in decreasing acidity and detoxifying the stomach and the liver.

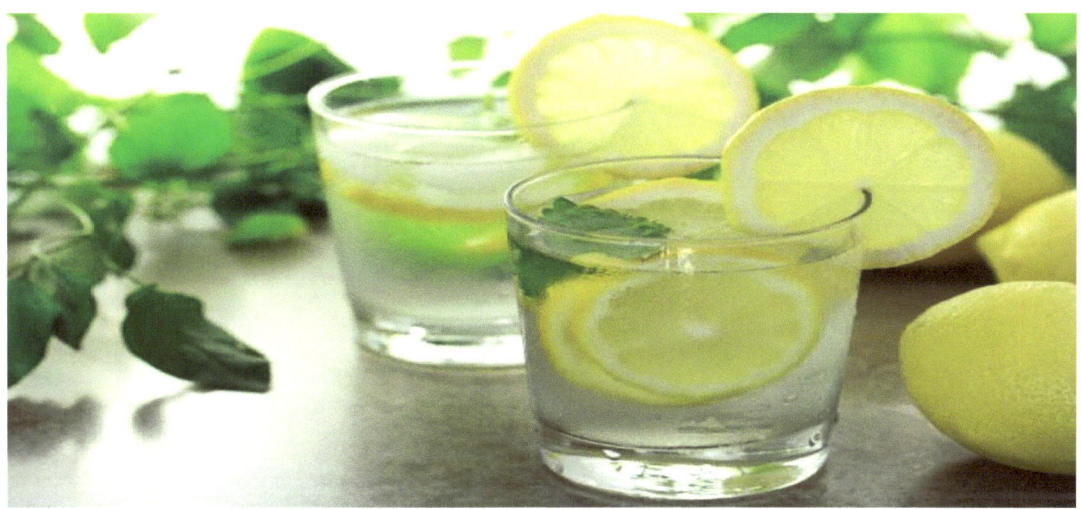

BLUEBERRIES

Blueberries are delicious little berries with a chock full of benefits. They help lessen pain by acting as a natural aspirin without any side effects! They also act as antibiotics and hence block bacteria, preventing infections. A full serving of berries can help in large amounts, in detoxifying the body since they are rich in phytonutrients called proanthocyanidins.

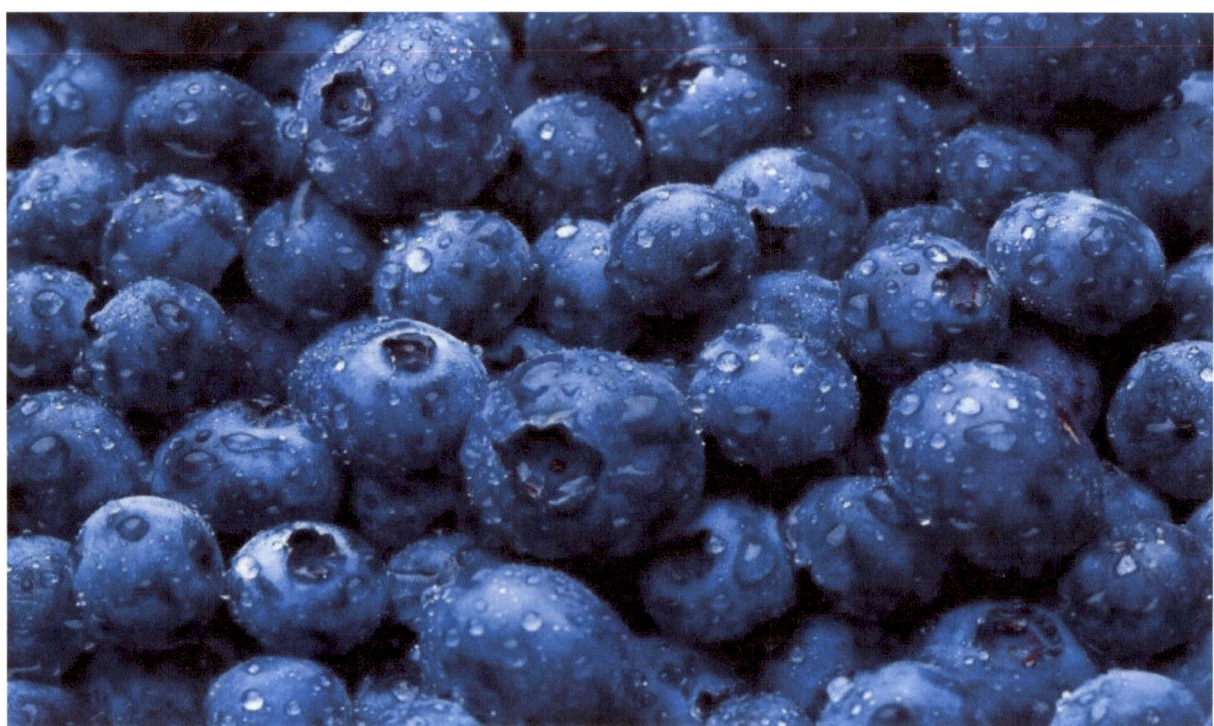

BASIL

Basil is also full of antioxidants, but it contains anti-bacterial properties additionally. As basil contains terpenoids, it is a good for detoxification and digestion. It helps the kidneys with their functions and also has anti-ulcer properties along with antimicrobial effects which act as a protection against yeast, bacteria, mold and fungi. Basil is often taken as one of the solutions for constipation. Also, basil can help viral infections due to its anticancer properties.

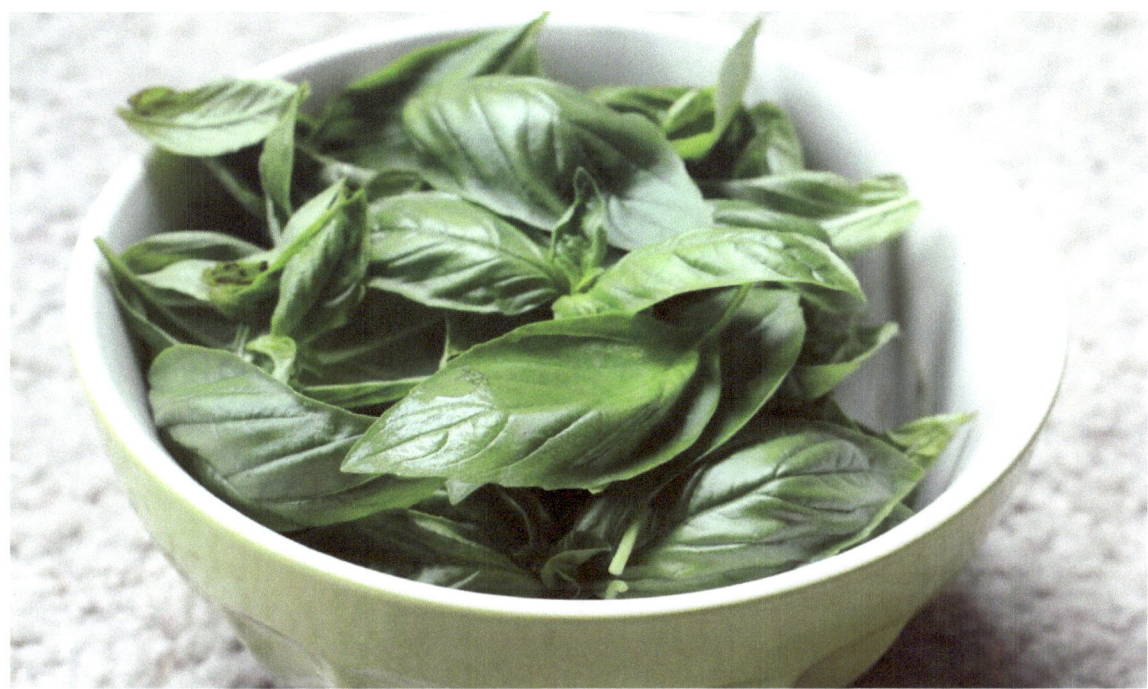

BEST SMOOTHIE RECIPES

All Berries Smoothie

Berries can just be your favorites when it comes to the most helpful smoothies. A berry smoothie can be one of the best fluids while and after detoxing because of all the fiber and antioxidants berries contain. A mixture of some berries can trigger the elimination of the harmful substances from your body. Here's the best recipe for the perfect blend of the berries.

Ingredients:

- 1 cup pure water

- 1/2 cup coconut milk

- 1 1/2 cups of mixture of berries like blueberries, raspberries and blackberries

- 1/8 cup rolled oats

Directions: Blend all the ingredients together until you reach an appropriate consistency of smoothie. The best part of this smoothie is that it doesn't require any preparations. Berries just need to be rinsed before blending.

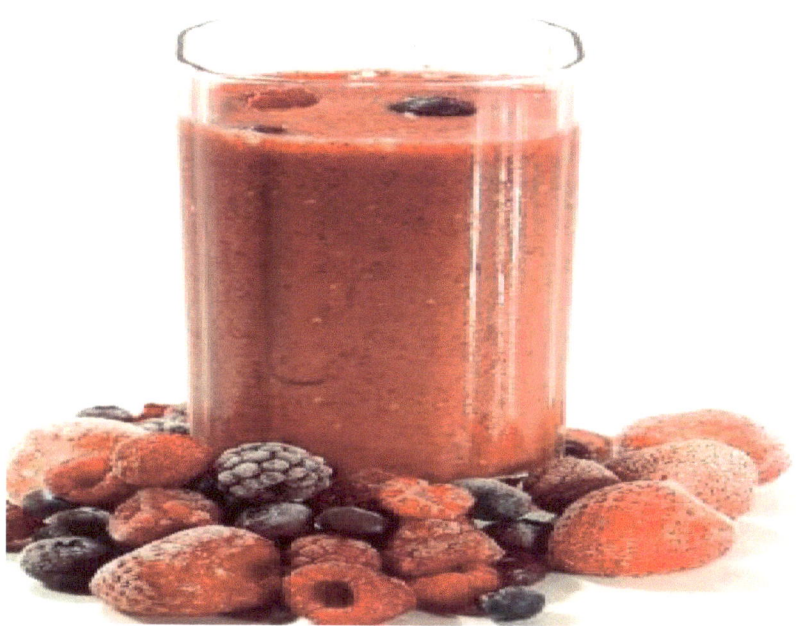

The Green Detox Smoothie

Ingredients:

- 1 medium-sized peeled banana

- 1 tablespoon chia seeds

- 1 peeled orange

- 1/2 peeled lime

- 1 small piece of grated ginger

- 8 ounce homemade almond milk or water

- 2 cups of kale or chopped dandelion greens

Directions: Soak the chia seeds 5 minutes before you start making the smoothie. Blend all the ingredients together except for dandelion greens. Blend it a few times, giving breaks in between. Then add the dandelion greens and blend for around 30 seconds until the blend looks creamy.

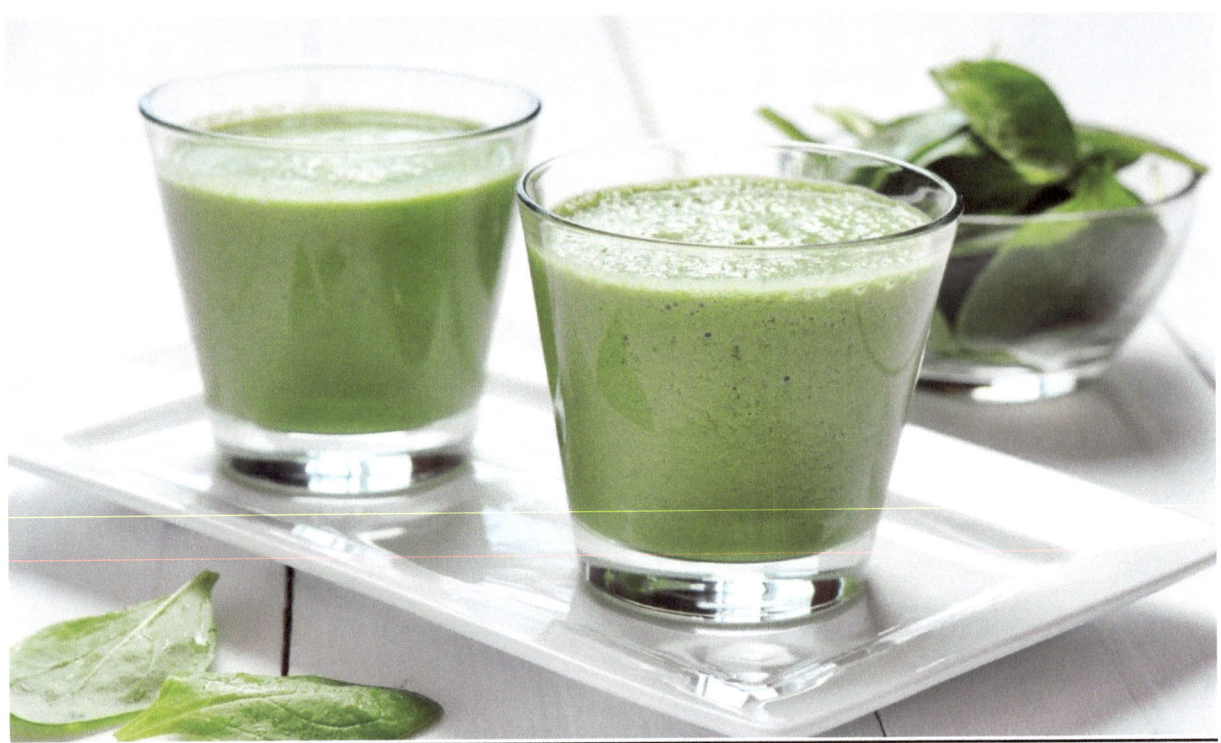

Kale-in Smoothie

Kale is one of the healthiest ingredients. One of the best ways to let your body benefit from it is making a tasteful smoothie. It does not require any preparations and you just need simple ingredients.

Ingredients:

- 1 cup of coconut water

- 1 handful of kale

- 1/2 apple

Directions: Baby kale is recommended to make blending easier, but if you take curly kale you must cut the stringy and hard ribs before you start blending. After this, just mix the ingredients and blend them all together until you see a smoothie texture.

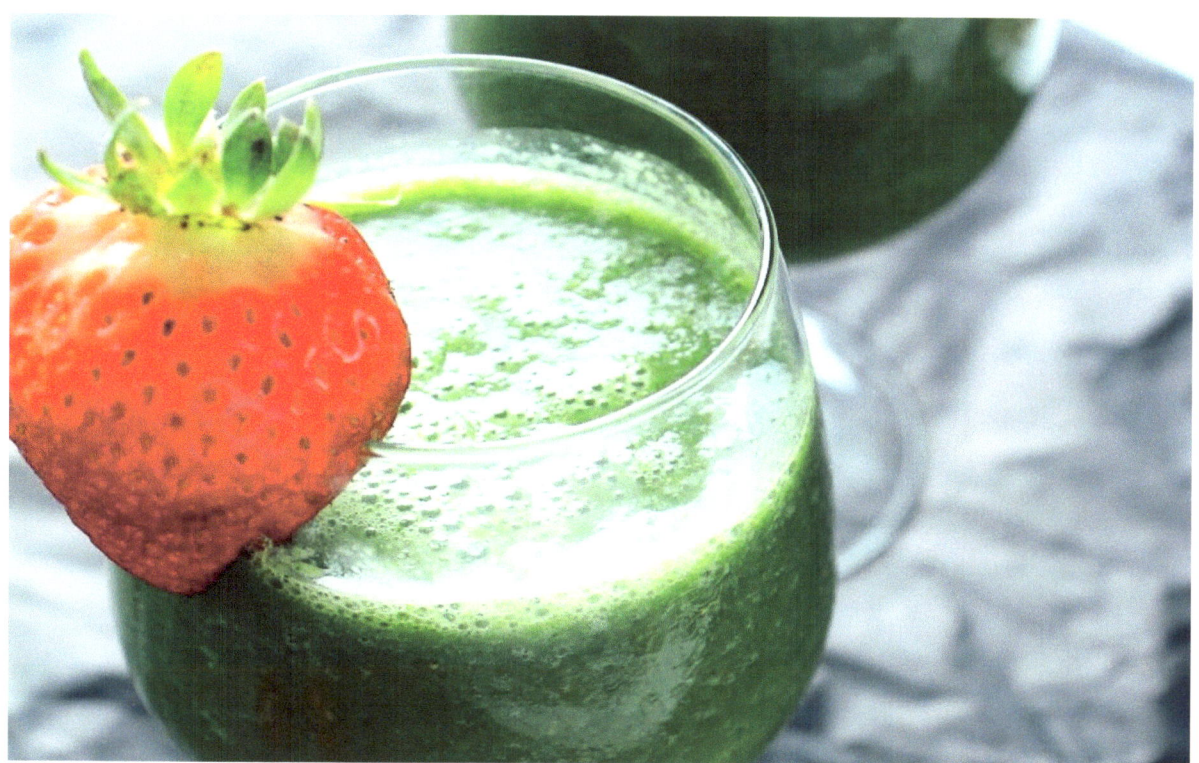

All-in-one Smoothie

This smoothie is full of healthy ingredients yet very light to drink. It's like getting all the useful nutrients in one glass.

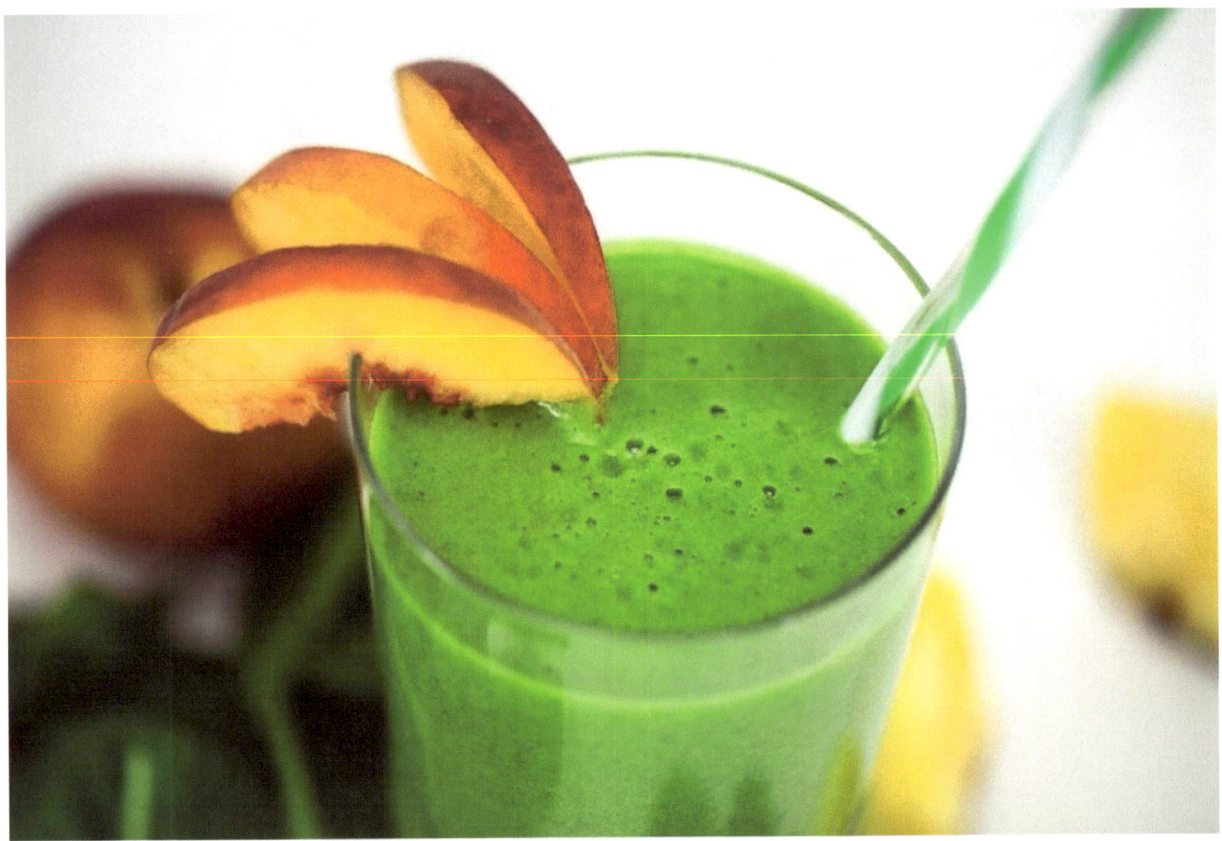

<u>Ingredients</u>

- 1 teaspoon bee pollen

- 3 leaves Cos lettuce

- 3 stalks of kale (use leaves only)

- 1 handful of blueberries

- 1 cup of coconut powder

- 1 teaspoon maca powder

- 1 teaspoon chia seeds

- 1 small banana (frozen recommended)

- 1 teaspoon hemp seeds

- 1 teaspoon spirulina

<u>Directions:</u> Just blend all of the ingredients together until they're smooth and ready for drinking.

CONCLUSION

A 5-day detoxification can wipe out the toxins from your body completely, if proper instructions are followed. However, what's more important is that you shouldn't change your lifestyle and get back to your eating habits directly after taking the program. Detoxification requires willpower more than any other thing. Controlling yourself, your cravings and your emotions is one big factor which will result in better overall health. You will need a lot determination because as mentioned earlier, you might actually feel worse during the process. Your physical and mental conditions will not get better until the process is over, and you pledge to follow some of the methods for the rest of your lives too.

It is also imperative to understand that you must not expect an overnight change in your body. The organs or the processes affected by the toxins we take with our food need some time to start functioning well again. This also explains that a change will not be observed, or will not retain if you start adding all those harmful, unnecessary substances in your body all over again.

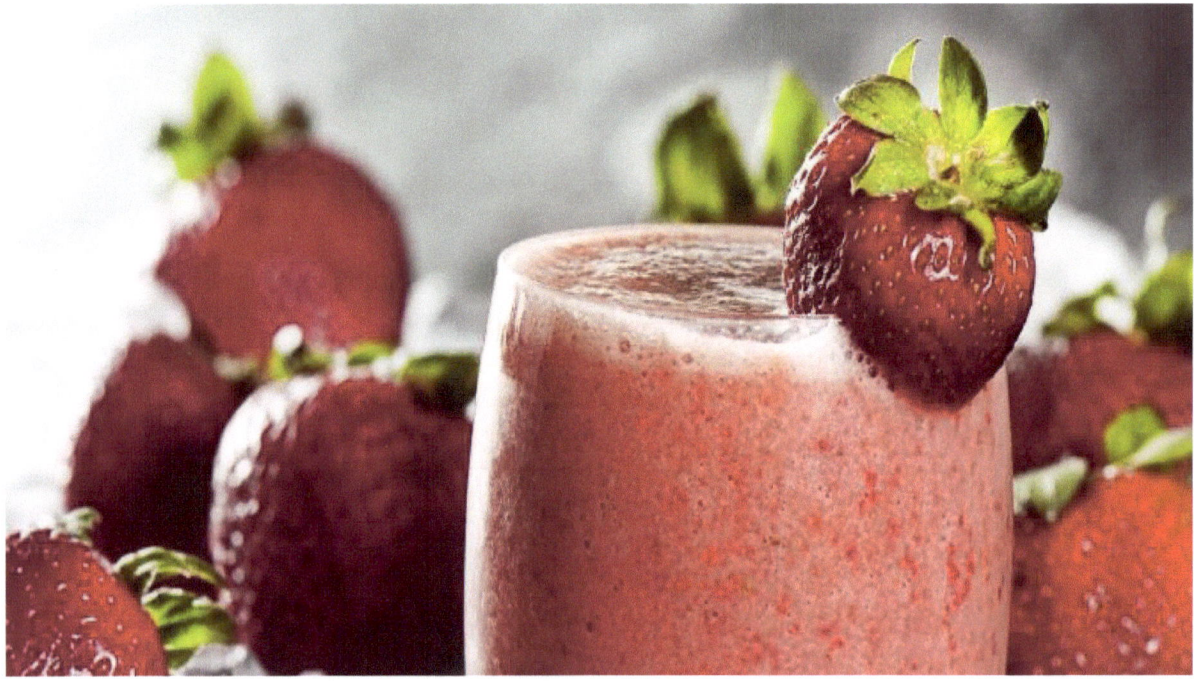

For more tips, recipes, and valuable information join us: Vegan Lifestyle and Soul Here!

Printed in the United States of America

First Printing, 2016

ISBN 9781523235933

Celeste2cs.com
6001 Argyle Forest Blvd Ste #21 PMB #373
Jacksonville, FL 32214

www.celeste2cs.com